THE SHADOW OF TREPIDATION

Reflections on caregiving during my
wife's battle with breast cancer

Keith T. Hardeman

outskirts
press

Dedication

I've faced two situations in my life when I knew precisely which people I could truly count on to help me when the chips were down: moving to a new residence, and living through my wife's cancer fight.

Though many friends, co-workers, and family members did so much for us throughout our terrible cancer ordeal, a few stood out and took their help to incalculable levels. This book is dedicated to them, and they are listed below, in no particular order.

Sam and Judy
Jim and Heather
Mark and Cinnamon
Bob and Lorena
Pat and Lucy (in Pat's loving memory)
Ginger and Jerry
Cliff
Sherry
Crystal
Holly
and especially Gordon

Shelley and I are indebted to each of you. You weren't just there when we needed someone. You went miles and miles above and beyond the proverbial call of duty. I don't know how we would have made our way through this mess without your help, your support, and your love.

Special thank-yous to our immediate family members are also in order. To Shelley's and my adult children Karen and Nick; to Shelley's parents Kenny and Linda and sister Teri; to my brother Jim and his wife Kris. You all were instrumental in constantly providing much needed emotional support from afar.

Table of Contents

Preface

Storytellers broaden our minds: engage, provoke, inspire, and, ultimately, connect us.

-Robert Redford

I never wanted to write this book.

I never wanted a story like this to tell.

Obviously, my retrospective wish is that my wife, Shelley, had never been diagnosed with breast cancer in the first place. I would give anything for her never to have suffered through the formidable, painful, and exhausting process of fighting cancer. And as the saying goes, I'd never even want my worst enemies to face the kind of extended physical and emotional agony she did. But since I obviously can't have that wish, I might as well try to put my story to good use in an attempt to help others as they begin traveling similar roads that Shelley and I have, to this point, mostly completed.

As a college professor of communication studies for some 40 years, I've long utilized the power of stories in my classrooms as a teaching strategy. In addition, a number of articles in various issues of *The Harvard Business Review* outline the benefits of storytelling. In one such work, Harrison Monarth explains that "a story can go where quantitative analysis is denied admission: our hearts."[1] This indicates to me that both the educational and business worlds recognize that storytelling is a valuable tool for teaching and learning in the real world. Listeners likely won't remember PowerPoint slides filled with lists of bullet-pointed statistics nearly as well as they'll retain an extended narrative, its plot, and its life lesson. I have a story, and it's not an easy one to tell. I also know that it's probably similar to experiences many people have to endure year after year.

Competent communicators will conduct an analysis of their intended audience in most every communication situation. The variety of classes I've taught have ranged from public speaking to interpersonal relationships, and organizational communication to journalism and public relations. To be patently effective, the sender of any message must consider who's receiving it, how it might be interpreted, and tailor it to their needs and comprehension level. It is, across the board, the most consistent lesson I teach to my students. Therefore, it is my intention to reach an audience of cancer fighters, caregivers, and those trying to help friends who are coping with this insidious disease.

I certainly could have used a book like this back in December 2017. As a new spousal caregiver, I wanted detailed stories from cancer fighters and survivors. I needed meticulous description from caregivers who'd been there before. As someone outside the medical community, I craved medical guidance in layman's terms so I could understand what was happening to my wife. I wanted to hear about how I could best serve her while her body was being demolished by the shock and awe of treatment. I needed to know how to take care of myself while caring for her. I sought predictability in coping with this ordeal.

But most of all, I needed a sense of big-picture realism regarding the physical and psychological ups and downs of cancer in order to help guide our hope of Shelley's full recovery. What I offer here is what I wished I'd had when I first started the coping and caregiving process.

According to the American Cancer Society, cancer diagnoses in the U.S. take place at a growing clip of over 1.8 million per year, or roughly one every 17.5 seconds.[2] One out of every three women and one out of every two men in this country will get cancer in their lifetimes.[3] Therefore, the odds of you or someone in your family getting cancer are fairly significant. That translates into the fact that there are a lot of people just like Shelley and me.

As a cancer fighter's husband, I was temporarily in a state of deep depression and overwhelming anxiety right after diagnosis. If my story can assist any present and future caregivers in pulling out of such mental anguish and forging roadways in coping and being effective in assisting their cancer fighters, I want it to do so. While some in the past thankfully have written about their cancer situations, new experiential accounts and perspectives still need to be shared. My goal with this book is to invite readers into our story – to feel emotionally what we felt.

I began writing about our journey on a healthcare social media site and then continued telling bits and pieces of our story by composing a couple of articles that were published in a wonderful and informative periodical called *Coping® with Cancer*. The magazine seems to be available in the waiting areas of many cancer clinics and hospitals. That's how I first came across it. After my articles were published, I was pleasantly surprised by several people around the country who graciously emailed me with appreciation, writing that my shared experiences were beneficial to them in their own cancer-coping worlds. Some of my colleagues and followers on social media went even further by suggesting I had a vital story to tell that might be appropriate for a book. But I resisted.

Let's face it, cancer stories are plentiful and are, perhaps, considered by some to be a dime a dozen. On the other hand, such vast numbers of stories keep piling up at an astounding rate – again, nearly two million each year – and each is unique to the individual patient and cancer family experiencing them.

As a requirement of my profession, I've been fortunate to be published with a number of peer-reviewed research articles in various academic journals, but they all reflect my educational training and professional expertise. This book, however, is significantly different. My purpose in sharing our story is based on trying to explain how cancer fighters feel when I've never been a cancer fighter. It's attempting to accurately and understandably describe medical procedures and information when I'm not a physician. It's examining psychological issues when I've had but one college freshman class in psychology. The only cancer expertise I can claim is in being a spousal caregiver. But I can't fully explain that without going into various realms of cancer fighting, medicine, and psychology and making sense of all of it so that readers new to the cancer experience might better understand what's happening as their journeys unfold.

Throughout this book, I've also tried to include appropriate rhetorical strategies from my academic expertise. I teach interpersonal communication skill units in empathy, semantics, listening, conflict resolution, and defensiveness restraint. Therefore, fortunately, it was often second-nature for me to pragmatically draw on this knowledge for, hopefully, more productive communication outcomes throughout Shelley's treatment. It is my humble wish that my descriptions of these interactional concepts and philosophies can be useful to other caregivers.

Overall, I want this work to be substantive while still a relatively quick read. Perhaps it can also serve as a good reference guide to which readers return if their own stories were the least bit commensurate to Shelley's and mine. I would never presume to speak for a cancer fighter. Or even for another caregiver. I speak only from my heart and with what wisdom I've gathered and can share from my own experiences and perspectives. Therefore, it is my sincere hope that this book can be valuable to those whose cancer stories are in motion or those that have yet to come.

Aside from friends and family listed in the book dedication, there are a few other people I wish to acknowledge and thank in bringing this project to fruition. First and foremost, I want to extend my endless gratitude to Karen Hay-Steuer who works as a writer, editor, translator and designer. Though we reside across the Atlantic Ocean from one another, Karen and I have maintained our close friendship that dates back to our college days at California State University, Long Beach in the late 1970s and early '80s. She not only put her editing and proof-reading skills to good use in reviewing this manuscript, she, more than anyone by far, kept encouraging me to continue and complete this work. Perhaps most importantly, she helped rebuild my occasion-ally waning confidence as she felt I truly had something important to say in the arena of cancer fighting and caregiving.

I offer my everlasting appreciation for the repeated contributions of my physician brother, Jim. He spent considerable time educating me and explaining the medical side of things at my level of compre-hension. His efforts were invaluable toward the completion of this work.

Next, I wish to thank Heather Gehlert, a dear friend who has openly shared with me her perspectives as a current breast cancer fighter and on caregiving. Her vivid descriptions allowed me to com-pare and contrast her journey with Shelley's, which hopefully added more to the accuracy in the way I have presented cancer survivor viewpoints. And, for clarification purposes, there are three breast cancer fighting/surviving Heathers referred to in this book.

I'm also grateful to some of my Westminster College colleagues, Professors Wayne Zade, David Collins, Linda Aulgur, Cliff Cain, Bob Cowles, and Tobias Gibson for their continued support throughout the process of my writing.

And, finally, to my late father and mother, Nicholas "Perk" Hardeman and Ada Mae Hardeman. I wish, somehow, you were still here to thank. The two of you will always be the most positively influential people in my life. Any successes I achieved in my profession took place in large part because I was able to stand on the shoulders of some very prominent individuals. Without the rock-solid foundation of values you taught me, those successes would have been far fewer in number. And the times when I've stood tallest were unquestionably because of the two of you. I miss you both tremendously.

CHAPTER 1

The Devastation and Fear of Diagnosis Day

It's just a shock. You go from one day everything being OK to your life being upside down.

-Amber Margarejo

"You have cancer."

Those three words are surely regarded as among the most frightening of verdicts anyone hears from a physician. The grim message is simple and to the point.

As a longtime *Seinfeld* fan, I often extend my vocabulary to include various terms and descriptors from that 1990s television sitcom. *High talker, refunding, shrinkage, mimbo, double-dipping,* and many other Seinfeldian vernacular examples routinely come to mind as I describe certain life situations. But when series co-star Julia Louis-Dreyfus announced her breast cancer diagnosis on September 28, 2017 via Twitter, her word choice, too, was unpretentious and haunting in reality: "1 in 8 women get breast cancer. Today, I'm the one."[4]

Cancer stories vary in outcome, but many of them begin similarly. A physician alerts you that a biopsy shows a malignant cell growth or tumor. Then multiple tests follow over the next seven to 10 days, which may provide answers and clarity about type, progression, stage, treatment, and survival. From that point, however, cancer fighters' stories can branch off into vastly different routes. Ultimately, the new cancer patient and family want those test results to reveal the single most important thing they can have at this time of darkness: a light of hope.

A great misconception about cancer is that it's one disease. It isn't. In fact it's many diseases.[5] The National Cancer Institute estimates there are over 100 types of cancer.[6] Though all cancers involve some type of uncontrolled cell growth, many of the similarities end there.[7] Cell structure, organ origination, and aggression levels can vary drastically.

And then there's metastasis, the deadly part of cancer. This is when it spreads, and in a stealth-like manner. Without any symptoms, one or a few cells from a malignant tumor can break off, travel through the bloodstream, and randomly attach to other organs in the body, where they recurrently divide to create additional life-threatening tumors that will likely lower one's survival chances. As author Clinton Crockett Peters so appropriately described, when cancer is growing inside one's body, it's like an internal "Frankenstein monster rampaging against its creator."[8]

Further mutations can occur when some malignancies develop resistances to various treatments, which can lead to the need for even more therapies. In addition, people can initially have nearly identical diagnoses and treatments, but completely different responses and outcomes to those medications.

As a professor in the humanities at Westminster College in Fulton, Missouri, I have no formal science or medical training whatsoever. However, I began my own obsession with cancer on January 9, 1992. On that terrible evening, my father passed away after his nearly six-and-a-half-year battle with non-Hodgkin's lymphoma. I felt the need to immerse myself in the war against cancer – not as a health care professional, of course, but as an advocate. I first needed to learn as much about the disease as I could. And I wanted to support community service organizations whose goals are to invest in cancer research, education, detection, treatment, patient rights, and, ultimately, to put themselves out of business by helping their funded researchers find the elusive cures.

In the ensuing years, I often donated money to the American Cancer Society (ACS), City of Hope, and the V Foundation. I gave presentations to various audiences about the need to escalate cancer funding through the ACS. And I repeatedly contacted my national representatives, urging them to significantly increase federal funding for cancer research and to pressure health insurance companies to cover preventative and early-detection cancer screenings. By 1998, I began annual participation in Relay For Life, the ACS's top fundraiser, and I personally raised $500 for that year's event in my father's honor and memory. But a family scare a couple of months afterward was so alarming that it caused me to ratchet up my efforts.

On a late summer day of that year, I was putting sunblock on my then five-year-old daughter when I noticed a couple of lumps under her arm. I took her to see our pediatrician soon after, and following several tests and a CT (computerized tomography) scan, he found a golf-ball-sized tumor in her abdomen. Based on the scan's visuals, he said, it could be benign or malignant, and that she would need surgery very soon to determine the next course of action. Our worst fear was that it was a neuroblastoma, which is a deadly nerve tissue cancer in children.

Five days later, the tumor was removed, and the pathology report eventually revealed it to be a benign ganglioneuroma. Clearly, we dodged a bullet. But that fear of "what if" motivated me to individually raise over $50,000 for the ACS over the next 14 years' of Relay events.

The perilous fellowship of cancer fighters and survivors is by no means an exclusive one. Lifestyle choices can certainly decrease one's odds of joining, but there is no sure-fire method to avoid the cancer club. Ever-growing research strongly suggests that many factors contribute to whether or not one's cancer is caught early, including socioeconomic divisions and access to adequate healthcare insurance and facilities. Quite regrettably, the ugly face of societal racism also seems to play a large role in detection delay, which ultimately lessens survival rates for some racial groups.[9] But cancer itself doesn't care about age, gender, sexual orientation, race, political views, religious beliefs, occupation, annual income, virtuosity, morality, or intelligence. Everyone – even those with the healthiest of personal habits – is susceptible.

A diagnosis is emotionally devastating. When it happens to you or someone close to you, it is quite normal be mired in fear, grief, and shock. During a 2019 *Good Morning America* interview with Robin Roberts, television game show host Alex Trebec revealed his own reaction to his stage 4 (IV) pancreatic cancer diagnosis: "I've had kidney stones, I've had ruptured discs, so I'm used to dealing with pain. But what I'm *not* used to dealing with is these surges that come on suddenly of *deep, deep sadness*, and it brings tears to my eyes."[10] I suspect most, if not all, newly diagnosed cancer patients and their families have no difficulty relating to that depiction.

I will always remember Wednesday, December 6, 2017 as one the saddest and most frightening days of my life. On that day, my beautiful wife, Shelley, became the one out of every eight women with a breast cancer diagnosis.

The fall semester was about to conclude. Christmas was on the horizon, and we were looking forward to our traditional family celebrations. But on Monday the 4th, Shelley confessed something she'd been keeping from me for the past week, mainly because she didn't think much of it at the time. She'd felt a lump in her right breast a couple of months earlier and finally went in to get it checked. She said that a precautionary biopsy had been done a few days prior. Results were expected on the morning of the 6th. Naturally, we were concerned, but Shelley, her mother, and her sister had all experienced breast cysts in their adult lives, and nothing ever came of them. And with the fact that Shelley's mammogram from just the previous week showed nothing out of the ordinary, both of us had good reason to believe that December 6 would come and go without incident.

We both went in to work early that morning, and I waited in my office for Shelley's call while quietly confident it would bring forth good news. At 8:42 am, my cell phone rang with Shelley on caller ID. When I answered, she let out a quiet, expressive sigh before saying anything, and I knew, at that very moment, our lives were about to change forever.

Shelley contained her emotion just long enough to blurt out, "It isn't good news. I have breast cancer." I quickly got up from my desk to shut my office door, and we both wept. Through her tears, she said, "I can't stay at work. [Co-workers] Sherry and Crystal are taking me home. Can you come home?"

"I'm leaving right now," I said. I quickly sent out a few obligatory, abbreviated emails to cancel afternoon classes and meetings, and then I discreetly exited through the back of my office building to my car. Now was definitely not the time to accidentally run into a student or colleague who might acknowledge me with a friendly smile and a greeting of "How's your day going, Keith?"

My 40-minute drive home seemed to take forever. Caught in a hyperventilating, panic-stricken daze, I had to consciously focus on driving safely. It wasn't easy, given the emotional circumstances. I pulled into the garage, ran up the stairs in the house, and stopped. Shelley was waiting by the living room couch. We stood still and locked eyes for a moment before we fell into each other's arms and emotionally fell apart. Our tight, sobbing embrace probably lasted a good 30 seconds before either of us could let go. Or speak. "They said I have lobular cancer," she revealed. I looked it up on the ACS website: invasive lobular carcinoma, a somewhat rare form of breast cancer compared with the more common ductal carcinoma.

We made an appointment with an oncologist, who would become a new main character in the story of our lives, and it was scheduled for the following morning at the Missouri Cancer Associates clinic. I guess we were lucky in one respect at least. Our long-time place of residence, the college town of Columbia, Missouri, home of the University of Missouri flagship campus, possesses state-of-the-art medical facilities that far belie its smaller size relative to large city medical access. CoMo, as it's affectionately nicknamed by many of its residents, has not one, but two regionally renowned cancer centers: Missouri Cancer Associates and Ellis Fischel. The trip to Shelley's appointments and treatments at MCA would only be a mere five miles from our home. We would later meet patients there, who needed to drive for several hours each way from all around the state and even some who came in from neighboring states.

Of course, our next emotional task on diagnosis day was having to alert family members: Our two adult children in Missouri, Shelley's parents and sister in Iowa, and my brother in California were first on the list. This was, obviously, sensitive news we couldn't just communicate impersonally through a text, email, or social media post. Some psychology experts believe that notifying others is among the most difficult parts of an initial diagnosis. Shelley and I would roundly agree with that assessment.

I made the first call. It was to Karen, our daughter who was now 24 years old and resided in Kansas City. I guess I felt the need to be strong for her, and I somehow held it together, though it meant being able only to talk in a very soft, monotone voice. She was silent at first and then sobbed uncontrollably. She frantically asked me the same questions about treatment and prognosis that I asked my own parents when my father was diagnosed back in 1985. And just like 32 years before, these were questions that wouldn't be answered for another week or two and only after a spate of test results. "I'll be home this weekend," she tearfully promised.

Shelley then phoned our son, Nick, a 21-year-old senior at Westminster College. She managed to catch him walking on campus between classes. Upon hearing the news, he literally fell to his knees as if the wind had been knocked out of him. "I'm coming home right now," he said.

The next call was to my older brother while he was at work as a physician in California. An internal medicine, pulmonary disease, and critical care specialist, he's scientifically objective and can be far less affected by the heat of a medical moment. But not this time. When I used "Shelley" and "invasive lobular carcinoma" in the same sentence, his reaction was a terse, whispered, "Oh… *fuck!*"

Predictably, Shelley's calls to her parents and sister didn't go well either. Both conversations included tears of desperation, with everyone naturally pressing us for details we couldn't yet provide.

These stressful interactions took everything out of us, emotionally and physically. Every call we made was more agonizing than the previous one. Our having to hear the initial reaction from each individual only rewound the pain process all over again. It was a one-time notification for them, but Shelley and I had to deal with it over and over. Undoubtedly, the enormity of this medical impact on our emotions was something we were not prepared to cope with at the outset. But, Jesus, who really is?

By the time Nick arrived home for the day, we simply couldn't summon the strength to make any more phone calls. While we were devastated by the news, there still was a familial comfort in the three of us being together for a few hours. But Nick's stay was temporary as he needed to return to campus for important pre-final-exam classes for the short remainder of the semester.

I then realized my sudden departure from work would not go unnoticed. I needed to alert several colleagues, close friends who, over the years, knew Shelley almost as well as they knew me. I also recognized that the moment we went public with this sensitive and delicate information, there would be no turning back. Our personal lives would be the focus of well-intentioned friends and colleagues trying to glean medical information from us and to somehow help us – whether we wanted the attention or not. Our privacy would be gone unless we set specific parameters. But the necessity for privacy versus the need for help is the great paradox as we communicate with others in these unfortunate situations. I quickly sent those colleagues an email explaining all that we knew, but with a caveat request:

> "For now, Shelley and I are still in the early stages of trying to sort things out and begin initial coping. The one thing we respectfully ask for, for at least the next 24 to 48 hours, is complete privacy. *Please do not call or text us.* I fully understand your need to convey your condolences, support, and well wishes, but we're under a lot of emotional strain in making the requisite calls to family. And we're still at the point where we're falling apart with each call. You may share this information with others, but please make a point to tell them not to contact us at this time. I will alert you when this communication moratorium concludes."

Both Karen and Nick came home two days later, and the four of us were able to spend part of the weekend for some much needed, private family grieving. A crisis can certainly bring out the best in families. Communication author Joseph A. DeVito describes family members' willingness to accept obligations toward one another: "… to offer comfort when family members are distressed, to take pleasure in their pleasures, to feel their pain, to raise their spirits."[11] Karen pointed out, in a complimentary tone, that it was the first time she'd ever seen me cry. "We're all in this together," I told her. "Right now we're going to support each other, and later we're going to celebrate our victories together."

A death sentence is frequently the conclusion many will naturally jump to when getting an initial cancer diagnosis. And for good reason. It's an utterly terrifying and emotionally overwhelming moment. Cancer is the number two killer in the U.S., right behind heart disease.[12] But diagnosis is only the beginning. We wanted immediate long-term answers. Everyone does. Unfortunately, it doesn't work that way. A crush of tests first had to be conducted. And only then would it begin to provide information to determine what potential outcomes we might expect. No question our fears grew by the hour. But so did our steely resolve to fight. And I soon crafted my own personal message to the beast:

"Go to hell, cancer. You took my father, my uncle, some of my favorite teachers, colleagues, students, and a few of my very best friends. But you're *not* going to take my wife. Certainly not without a fight. Like the irredeemable coward you are and always have been, you deviously sneaked up behind us. You gained strong momentum in quietly assembling vast numbers of well-placed microscopic troops while we weren't looking. And no question we are definitely afraid in that we already know your dastardly plan. But you're in our crosshairs, now. We'll have our own army: a group of oncological experts who will inflict mortal damage to you on multiple levels. They're going to bombard you with lethal poison. They'll engage you in hand-to-hand combat with razor-sharp scalpels to cut the life right out of you. And they'll probably utilize nuclear warfare in frying you with intense, repeated radiation. Lord knows we'll get beaten up a lot in the process. But if it's a fight to the death you want, you've got one. You think we won't weather this storm? You gutless asshole, my wife *will be* the storm."

CHAPTER 2

Hurry Up and Wait!

Not everything that is faced can be changed. But nothing can be changed until it is faced.

-James Baldwin

Upon hearing our diagnosis news, Shelley and I overtly hoped for the best, but we quietly dreaded the worst. These reactions were triggered not just by the initial finding, but perhaps more so by the vast fear of the unknown. Questions pervaded our every thought: How far advanced is her cancer? What is the prognosis? How difficult will treatment be? Will she even survive? These questions repeatedly played themselves out in our minds, and we would soon pose them to our new oncologist. When I say "we," it is to state unequivocally that, as Shelley's husband and cancer caregiver, I saw this as a team effort. The one thing I promised her was that, if at all possible, I would set up my work schedule to allow me to join her at every physician's appointment and treatment she had. She would never be alone, as I'd stay by her side, every step of the way.

It was a seasonably cold December 7 morning as we pulled into the Missouri Cancer Associates parking lot for the first time. We walked in, approached the front desk, and Shelley was handed a clipboard with an abundance of paperwork to fill out. The clinic was thoroughly adorned with Christmas decorations. There was a part of me that was relatively annoyed by the tinsel, trees, wreaths, twinkling lights, and ornaments, since I was most certainly not in any kind of cheerful holiday mood. I even heard several employees happily wishing a few of the patients to "have a Merry Christmas," as they were leaving. "Merry fucking Christmas, indeed," I very softly and sarcastically mumbled to myself.

Shelley was expressionless as she dutifully filled out every section of her medical history and insurance information. The faces of others in the waiting area seemed equally blank, if not hopeless. It was easy to differentiate some of the cancer patients from their accompanying caregivers. The frail bodies, the thinning hair, hats and turban-like head coverings, and the ashen complexions were clear giveaways of veteran cancer fighters. But given our respective appearances, I wondered at that moment if others could tell between Shelley and me who the cancer fighter was.

After Shelley completed the paperwork, we were sent to the exam room to meet our oncologist. We sat in complete silence until Dr. Makarian walked in. She introduced herself and was very objective and business-like. She asked Shelley a few questions about family medical history and how she was feeling before commencing the physical exam.

"It feels like about two centimeters," she said, from her manual estimate of the tumor size. "We will need to schedule a PET (positron emission tomography) scan and an MRI (magnetic resonance imaging) to determine the actual size of the tumor and stage of your cancer." When we asked for more specifics, all she could offer, at that point, were speculations of best- and worst-case scenarios. She discussed possible treatments and, as we anticipated, said Shelley would likely have chemotherapy, radiation, and some type of surgery, whether it was a lumpectomy or mastectomy.

This was a common theme we noticed among the various physicians with whom we consulted at the outset: If this, then this. However, if that, then that. It didn't help when we were hell-bent on knowing everything *now*; there was no fast-forward button to press or spoiler-alert to read. We had to be patient as this journey could only play itself out in real time. Dr. Makarian took special care in explaining to us the reasons for the perceived delay. Her plan was to get Shelley started with chemotherapy in two weeks, on December 21. Of course, we wanted things to begin sooner than that. But in addition to the PET scan and MRI, a lot had to happen before then in preparation:

- The biopsy needed to be checked for a week or so to see how it would respond to prospective chemotherapies and hormonal treatments. I actually thought this was fascinating that they could test, in advance, for the most effective, individualized way to treat Shelley's specific cancer in what seemingly amounted to microscopic target practice for the lab and oncologist.
- Shelley would need an echocardiogram to determine whether her heart was strong enough to tolerate the harsh, noxious chemicals of the treatment.
- Since she had terrible veins for blood tests, Shelley agreed it would be best to have a chemotherapy port surgically installed in her chest, on the left side, opposite the tumor in her right breast.

"Look, I *know* that everyone wants to get started immediately, but whatever stage you're at will not change at all in the next two weeks," Dr. Makarian assured us. "It's far better for us to learn as much as we can about biopsy reaction, tumor size, and stage at the outset. It's best to start treatment a little later and get it right than to start too soon and get it wrong, which could have devastating consequences," she added. Suffice to say that we connected quickly with Dr. Makarian and her nurse, Ashley. We were very glad to have both of them on our oncology team.

When we weren't in hospitals or clinics for testing, Shelley and I read up on her type of cancer, and even some blogs and articles on how people cope with the shocking news at the outset. One person wrote, "…there's actually nothing more brave than being able to show how afraid you are of something that is scary. Or how sad you are about something that is really sad. To me, that's real bravery."[13] We hoped that was true. Because we both were very afraid. And incredibly sad.

While we tried to maintain overall privacy at the start, we did actively seek out a few friends who had experienced or were currently enduring cancer and its treatment. We called Jim and Heather as well as Pat and Lucy for advice on initial coping. If anyone could empathize with our new roles, they could. Heather had persevered through breast cancer several years prior and was still on her daily adjuvant[i] tamoxifen treatment, while Pat was in a long-term, Herculean battle with leukemia and metastatic prostate cancer. Jim and Lucy were their respective, loving, spousal caregivers. Shelley had a number of conversations with Heather regarding treatment and side effects. I was interested in how Jim and Lucy managed the psychological struggles of coping with the diagnosis and of caregiving.

Jim was very empathetic. "I'll never forget the overwhelm you're feeling right now," he said. "At the outset, don't even try to understand everything that's happening. It's absolute *chaos*. It doesn't seem like it now, but it will come to you, and, believe it or not, the 'new normal' will at least be predictable, unlike what's going on right now."

Heather thoughtfully told me, "I know that my breast cancer diagnosis and treatment was as hard on Jim in every way but physically as it was on me. So, please know that we are here for you as much as we are for Shelley."

---

i   Adjuvant treatment refers to continuing or secondary therapy after the original chemo, surgical, and/or radiation regimen has concluded. It is used for the purpose of subduing potential cancer recurrence.

"You'll probably cry. A lot," said Lucy. "It's what Pat and I did. So don't be ashamed of it. Just accept it."

"I think the first time you hear 'cancer' about yourself or a loved one, it is shock," Pat added. "But given all the treatments available today, one has to be optimistic."

Both couples got their treatments at MCA, and all four individuals were extremely complimentary of the care they received. Lucy said that she and Pat "could not be more pleased with the talent of his oncologist, radiologists, staff, and all. Such a caring and comforting place." "I promise they will take *good* care of you," Jim added. These discussions were *very* helpful in a vicarious way, but they still didn't assuage the totality of our fears. I guess acceptance would just have to come bit by bit as we experienced that new normal ourselves.

Waiting was not only torturous for us, but also for our family and close friends who felt as helpless as we did. Right after we returned home from MCA, I sent another email alerting those friends that our post-diagnosis communication hiatus concluded.

Immediately, they began sending messages, pining to know what, if anything, they could somehow do to help. But at that moment, there was just nothing anyone could do. We had to wait at least for the initial test results. Our friends' sustained contact was a bit overwhelming, at times. We soon realized we had to figure out a communication strategy that could keep everyone apprised and up to date while maintaining the privacy and separation we often needed. Phone calls were *so* draining; they had to be reserved just for the very closest of friends and family members. But more public means of reaching the masses through electronic channels seemed to invite other inherent problems. Email, texting, and social media would still facilitate individual responses, many of which would likely be pressing us with even more questions that we weren't prepared to answer. While Shelley has a social media account (I do not), she wanted, instead, to reserve it for more breadth of life occurrences than focusing on her cancer.

Heather helped us solve the communication problem. She alerted us to a social-media health-crisis web site called CaringBridge (www.caringbridge.org) that she used as an effective method for informing everyone about her own cancer journey. The site makes it easy to update interested parties on one's condition, to alert them when specific help is needed, and it allows followers to offer their support and encouragement while maintaining the family's privacy. I soon opened a CaringBridge account, and it wasn't long before I began posting updates. I quickly learned that another benefit of using this site and platform was that writing posts actually turned out to be quite cathartic in the psychology of my own coping process.

Before chemo began, Shelley and I decided to spend as much special, couple time together as we could. While we still could. About all I could tell myself at that point was an endless series of clichés about taking things one day at a time and living for today. It may have sounded like bullshit trivial platitudes to others, but those thoughts seemed to carry us along, at least at the start of everything. We did our best to live in the present. Before treatment, Shelley actually felt physically fine, so we decided to have several spur-of-the-moment dinner dates.

One of those dinners out took place on Sunday night, December 10. We went to a local Mexican diner, and Shelley and I were literally the only patrons in the restaurant. As we neared the end of our meal, a young family of four walked in and was brought to an adjacent table. The parents and their small children were bundled up in winter coats, scarfs, mittens, and stocking caps before removing them to sit down.

And when the mother took off her own cap, she revealed a completely bald scalp. We suspected that she might be a cancer fighter, and we inconspicuously watched everyone in the family interact with her as if her appearance were completely normal. Which, to them, it obviously was. She smiled a lot and seemed to really enjoy this time with her family. I then looked back at Shelley and quietly said to her, "OK. That's an affirmation that life continues through the cancer fight." She nodded in agreement.

After dinner, we drove around Columbia and looked at Christmas lights. And we talked, very frankly, about the realities of the situation we faced, about the unconditional love we had shared as a couple for nearly 30 years, and about how we would be there to hold the other up during this terrible battle. We knew that Shelley's role in the ordeal would be the most difficult in coping with the disease and its prospective physical horrors of chemo: the terrible nausea, the hair and weight loss, the hit-by-a-truck fatigue. And we also knew (as our good cancer-fighting friends had previously pointed out) that the second most difficult role would my caregiving, as I could only watch the person I loved most on the planet suffering when I'd be helpless to do much of anything but be there with her.

We had 10 or so nights like that, and we used them very, very wisely. We even spent some time putting up our tree and a few decorations. Since Karen and Nick were going to be home for Christmas, we didn't want our house to be completely barren during the holiday season.

In the meantime, our friends and colleagues were incredibly generous. Some began to surprise us with prepared meals. Others delivered gift cards to various restaurants. At a time when neither Shelley nor I felt much like eating or even making the effort to cook, those wonderful people constantly reminded us that we were not alone. It seems that we live our friendship lives gearing ourselves up for horrible situations like this. They did not disappoint. We knew they were hurting a lot too.

As part of cancer's new series of psychological ups and downs, Tuesday, December 12 was one of our more emotionally difficult days, because we were faced with some of the graphic, physical realities that potentially awaited us. We had an appointment consult with the surgeon, Dr. Peterson, who would be removing the tumor. But again, until the PET scan was conducted to reveal specifics (and, ultimately, the conclusion of chemotherapy months later), we wouldn't know if Shelley would be having a lumpectomy (tumor removal), a mastectomy (removal of the breast), or a double (bilateral) mastectomy in the event the cancer had also spread into her left breast.

It was a lot to digest, substantively and emotionally. Minutes after that appointment was the consult with the plastic surgeon. Since Shelley was facing the possibility of losing one or both breasts, we listened to options about reconstructive surgery, which was also described in detail (including explicit photos) as what could be a long and sometimes uncomfortable process. She was only 52. If breast removal were necessary down the line, she would eventually need to come to grips with having only one or no breasts at all. The prospect of upper body disfigurement as a treatment only enhanced her anxiety.

Just as Alex Trebec explained with his own reactions to his cancer ordeal, I was repeatedly hit by surges of sadness. And fear. For those two weeks between diagnosis and the start of chemo, I didn't eat or sleep much. And I'm not embarrassed to disclose that the emotional trauma was clearly getting the best of me. I kept imagining life without Shelley. As my friend Jim had warned, it was utter chaos under the information landslide during numerous doctors' visits and tests. All of which provided emotionally charged, often delayed medical information that we sometimes didn't understand. Everything was horribly new while we faced the terrifyingly unknown. There were times I'd be fine, and then, without warning, it just hit me and started all over again. I think it's safe to say that cancer families are far more sensitive at this time and often react emotionally to even the most innocuous of things people say. And that's because, as journalist Alexandra Gloriososo insightfully wrote about her own diagnosis, "…whatever cancer isn't doing to [the] body, it's definitely doing to [the] mind."[14]

How does one cope at the very outset? There is no easy answer. Upon Jim's suggestion, we stopped trying to make sense of everything that was taking place, because there was simply too much to absorb at once, with too many scenarios to consider. In this new crisis world, one must be patient and prepared to wait. A lot. As I've stated, we went from appointment to appointment, rushing to arrive on time and then waiting. From the 7th to the 20th of December, we had almost daily appointments and tests. But much of it was spent in arduous waiting. Waiting to assemble the oncology team, as we needed consults with each of them individually. Waiting for physicians to get us into their already bursting-at-the-seams schedules. Waiting in clinics. Waiting for test outcomes on the biopsy. Waiting for the PET scan and MRI, and waiting for radiologists to evaluate and give us those results. And knowing that the waiting was necessary and inevitable still didn't make it any easier to experience. But get results, we finally did, on Friday, December 15. And not quite the ones we'd hoped for.

Cancer is normally staged at one through four (I-IV).[ii] The TMN system is usually used to determine stage of breast cancer: tumor size, metastasis extent, and how many lymph nodes are affected.[15] Generally, stage I cancer means it's been discovered very early, prior to any evident progression of the disease to the lymph nodes or other organs. Survival rates tend to be higher if it's caught at this point. Stage IV means it has spread, considerably, and the survival rate is significantly lower. There are also increments between stages designated by letters: Breast cancer typed at stage IIB probably has a slightly larger tumor and/or a bit more reach into surrounding lymph nodes than IIA. But it's still short of stage III progression. It's also important to note that the staging process isn't always foolproof since scans can't detect microscopic development. Therefore, some cancers that are initially

---

ii   According to the National Breast Cancer Foundation, there is also a stage 0 which can be detected as abnormal cells prior their becoming invasive in nature.

determined to be stage I may already have individual metastasizing cells missed by the scans that end up creating new tumors as a result.

Shelley's initial ultrasound, biopsy, and manual touch led to an estimate of a two-centimeter tumor, with it having spread to two lymph nodes. Our hope was that it was only at stage II. But the PET scan revealed that the tumor was more than three times that size – seven centimeters – and that it was more advanced than originally thought. Her cancer had invaded at least five lymph nodes. We were at stage IIIA. It apparently hadn't metastasized beyond the nodes, so I guess that part was "good." But it had spread more than we'd hoped. Shit.

In addition to becoming acclimated to all the waiting, my physician brother warned us of something that we'd already begun to figure out: the need to prepare for many emotional vicissitudes. He suggested very early in the game that this was going to be a marathon, and that it was best not to let ourselves get too depressed if things temporarily went south or too giddy in response to what may seem like positive information. He also wanted to give us legitimate hope by adding that medical technology has made some incredible oncological advances in the last couple of decades, or so. Breast cancer research, in particular, he said, has moved at almost warp speed. But cancer also has a historical penchant for figuring out ways to counteract some of the therapies. It's often a chess match between the disease and the physicians. And, unfortunately, it was physically painful for Shelley since the chessboard is the body of the cancer fighter.

In all, the new knowledge was an out-and-out bludgeoning of sometimes incomprehensible medical reports containing the most serious of outcomes and scenarios. And it was December. Medical professionals, who are also people with lives outside their work commitments, were understandably wishing to spend time with their families to celebrate the winter holidays. Moreover, we had to deal with an unintentional "left hand not quite knowing what the right hand is doing" scheduling snafu. Hospital tests and procedures conducted in different departments must take place in a specified order and time frame. And one department needs to be clearly aware of the other when this happens.

Dr. Makarian outlined the chemo regimen. The first four treatments would be a toxic cocktail of doxorubicin and cyclophosphamide, which are the respective generic names for Adriamycin® and Cytoxan®. Together, we knew them as the AC treatment. Adriamycin is known among medical personnel and chemotherapy patients as "The Red Devil." In addition to its bright red color, it is a horrible chemical agent that causes a number of nasty side effects. Together with Cytoxan, severe nausea and vomiting, diarrhea, drastic fatigue, potential heart damage, and hair loss were possible, and probably inevitable. These treatments would be administered every two weeks for four cycles.

At the completion of AC, the chemo schedule and type would change to 12 weekly rounds of Taxol® (paclitaxel), an effective follow-up chemo which tends to have less severe, but different and bothersome, side effects. If all went well, Shelley could complete her chemotherapy on May 4, 2018. But we couldn't get too far ahead of ourselves.

Not only are the side effects sometimes intolerable, chemotherapy crushes one's immune system. And in December, we were headed full steam into cold and flu season. We would be incredibly fortunate if we never had to miss or delay any of the 16 scheduled rounds over the course of the next four and a half months. But then surgery and radiation would follow in June and July. Our best-case scenario would be that she'd beat it and be completely finished sometime in late summer or early fall of 2018. Of course, it would likely take months – maybe years – of healing beyond the blitzkrieg of treatment before her body might feel normal, again. Assuming that one day it would. The worst-case scenario? Well, we tried our best not to allow ourselves to think in those terms at all during December.

Once we had the results of the scan, it was time to get the echocardiogram done and the port installed before chemo could commence. That year Christmas was on a Monday, which meant Missouri Cancer Associates wouldn't be open over the extended weekend. Therefore, a lot was being squeezed in during a short amount of time. Getting appointments lined up before Christmas proved to be a bit difficult. The port surgery was already scheduled for 1:00 pm on Wednesday, December 20 with the first chemo planned for Thursday, the 21st. But neither of these would take place without the echo, and we were still waiting on an appointment time for that.

When we were notified that the echo would be at 11:45 the morning of the 20th, Shelley suspiciously asked, "Are you sure that will be enough time for me to get to my 1:00 surgery?" "Oh, absolutely," said the receptionist. "You should be finished with the echo by 12:30 at the latest. The surgery department is literally 100 feet from cardiology."

Because of the 1:00 pm surgery, Shelley had been instructed not to eat after midnight the previous night. We arrived at the hospital in plenty of time for the 11:45 echo appointment. Unfortunately, as often happens in the medical-appointment world, they were running late, and things didn't get started until about 12:05.

It didn't matter.

About 10 minutes into the echocardiogram procedure, Shelley's phone rang. When I pulled it out of her purse and saw the hospital on her caller ID, I was a bit puzzled as I answered. It was the surgery department. "Uh, was Shelley coming in to surgery, today?" a woman politely asked. "We have a two-hour surgery prep time and were expecting you to be here by 11 am for the 1:00 surgery."

Unfortunately, neither department relayed that useful information to us as they were setting up the schedules. The appointment-makers made the unintentional omission errors, and we paid the price. Because of that necessary prep time, Shelley's surgery didn't start until after 3:00 pm. And, of course, she hadn't eaten since the night before. She was even more famished prior to the port installation.

With the fresh wound of a tube surgically implanted in her upper left chest, that night Shelley was very uncomfortable in terms of sleeping. She had to sleep on her back, which she was not accustomed to doing. When she would momentarily drift off, she was immediately awakened by a stabbing pain whenever she began to change sleeping positions. It was a very restless, if not pretty much sleepless, night for both of us.

CHAPTER 3

Chemotherapy – The First Is Often the Worst

This is my chemo mug. And I will smash it into a thousand pieces when this is all over.

-printed on a coffee mug sold on Amazon.com

You probably know of someone with cancer who has undergone the dreadfully unpleasant experience of chemotherapy treatment. Standard chemo is toxic poison. For the most part, it is engineered to target rapidly growing cells such as cancer. But it doesn't differentiate between malignant cells and normal cells. Healthy hair follicles, fingernails and toenails, and cells lining the gastrointestinal tract also reproduce quickly, and it makes sense that chemo would hit those areas hard as well. Hence, hair loss, nail discoloration and damage, and severe nausea are primary and common side effects of this chemical treatment that many cancer fighters experience. Since standard chemo can't be specifically aimed to avoid noncancerous cells, it goes through the entire body. And it affects everything. Healthy cells are pushed to their limits in fighting back, and fatigue simply takes over. Different types of chemo can have varying effects. Some of them may be less intense, but distastefully difficult, nonetheless.

Likely no two people react to chemo quite the same way. On one of our nurse's recommendations, Shelley decided very early in the game that one thing she wouldn't read up on were individual horror stories about chemo. Since those who write about their own experiences on the internet often tend to describe the worst of the worst, she was concerned about the potential mind-game effects such testimonials might create. "Trust me when I say that *nothing* about chemo side effects is pleasant," Shelley would later tell me. "But I wasn't always affected the way others were."

Throughout her months of treatment, we did participate in many story exchanges among cancer fighters in the infusion room. As we heard about each unique cancer story, descriptions of chemo reactions seemed to be every bit as individualized. Just as there is a multitude of cancer types, there are many kinds of chemo, and their specific use depends on what type of cancer is being treated as well as its stage and location. One's age, overall health, and other various personal factors such as heredity are also taken into consideration.[16]

With her infusion port freshly installed the previous afternoon, Shelley's first Adriamycin/Cytoxan (AC) chemo treatment was scheduled for 8:00 am on Thursday, December 21. We arrived at Missouri Cancer Associates at 7:50 and soon went to the nurse's station to have her blood drawn to determine blood cell counts. We quickly learned the results were good, and our next stop was the infusion room.

When we sat down at a therapy station, a relatively young and very upbeat chemotherapy nurse named Lindsay approached us. She saw on Shelley's chart that this was her first treatment. Nurse Lindsay sat down with us, carefully explained everything that was about to happen, and did so in understandable terms. Shelley would be getting anti-nausea drugs in addition to the chemo, and the entire process would take about two hours. Lindsay told us that we'd also be prescribed some strong, oral anti-nausea meds, Zofran® (ondansetron) and Compazine® (prochlorperazine), to pick up at our pharmacy on our way home. We cautiously hoped this would fend off what we feared were the inevitable vomiting sessions.

"OK, then let's do this," Shelley said, obviously wanting to get it over with sooner than later. All we needed, now, was the chemo.

"We're ready to go, but I'm afraid we can't start just yet," Lindsay said, apologetically. "We can't start the infusion until your echocardiogram is approved by a cardiologist, and we're still waiting on that. Hopefully, it'll be soon."

Ah. I'm sure I must have mentioned something about waiting in the previous chapter.

We sat and waited there at the station. And waited. And waited. At 9:15 I walked over to Nurse Lindsay and asked if this would be much longer.

"I'm so sorry for this," she said with an exasperated look. "I've called twice, and the cardiologist on call hasn't gotten back to us, yet." By 10:30, both Shelley and I were admittedly having some difficulty containing our frustration. But we were very pleased to see that Lindsay seemed equally frustrated. I listened in to what was at least her third phone call to the hospital cardiology department. She was polite. And she was firm. "Would you please tell the doctor that she's been sitting here for nearly three hours, and ask him to prioritize her?" I was impressed as hell with her tone and advocacy.

Throughout the wait, we often heard the sound of electronic bells going off and didn't quite know what to make of them. "That signifies that the patient has completed infusion," Lindsay explained. We were almost jealous that a number of cancer fighters, who arrived after we did, were finishing while we waited just to get started. But then again, knowing the potential side effects that would likely follow, we weren't all *that* keen on starting, either.

In retrospect, I have absolutely no doubt that all players involved in this medical sequence were doing their level best. It wasn't as if the cardiologist didn't have other important patients. And we obviously wanted him to go through Shelley's echo results with meticulous care to be certain her heart could endure the stress of the chemotherapy cocktail.

At 11:07, Lindsay walked over while holding a few infusion bags, and each was filled to capacity. "I'm *so* sorry for the wait, you guys," she said in a contrite tone. "But your echo results just came in, they're good, and we're ready to go."

"Thank you for all you're doing, here," I responded with equal contrition. "I'm sorry if we seem frustrated. This has just been a rather difficult couple of weeks."

Shelley momentarily grimaced as Lindsay inserted a needle into the skin flap covering the port. The drip began. "I have to check on other patients, but I'll be back soon to see how you're doing," Lindsay said.

Nurse Lindsay is a model of what I'm certain all nurses aspire to be. She's knowledgeable, caring, empathetic, and she listens very well. She takes time to connect with patients and their caregivers during the chemotherapy processes. And we definitely connected with her. As I observed other patients and their respective nurses in the infusion room, very similar interactions were taking place. If we *had* to go through this horror, we were glad to be in the care of Missouri Cancer Associates.

Our breast-cancer-survivor friend, Heather, was gracious enough to bring us lunch during the drip. We were concerned about nausea, but Lindsay told us Shelley had been loaded up with Zofran and Compazine, and that, if she could possibly keep it down, nourishment was important at this time. We ate well, and then our own bell finally rang as we finished a little after 1:00 pm. We stopped at the pharmacy for her oral meds and arrived home at about 1:30. Shelley sat on the couch. "I don't want to speak too soon," she said, "but I actually feel pretty good."

Quite sadly, she spoke far too soon.

Within three hours, everything turned perfectly horrible. In spite of taking her nausea medication beforehand, by 4:30 pm, Shelley was violently throwing up for the next 90 minutes. To the point of utter exhaustion. Her facial complexion was positively white. She could barely hold her head up over the toilet during this seemingly endless bout of brutal vomiting. Those who have endured stomach illness from the flu, gastrointestinal problems, or the consumption of too much alcohol likely could not fully appreciate the sheer rage of chemotherapy's ghastly abdominal exit power. All I could do was watch her, hold her, feel her convulse, and listen to her suffer. She managed to take a Compazine in between sessions, but regurgitation actions were already in full swing, and she could not keep it down.

The vomiting finally ended at 6:00 pm. Shelley couldn't even stand up without my help. I held her tightly and slowly walked her to the living room sofa, which was the closest place for her to lie down. She simply collapsed. I placed a cold washcloth on her forehead and a bucket near her face in case the sickness resumed without warning. She was fast asleep within 90 seconds. With one exception when I needed to wake her up briefly, she was completely out for about four hours.

The exception was an anticipated phone call from Karen that came at 9:15. Even in the middle of this horrible episode, something good still managed to take place. She called to tell us that her long-time boyfriend, Jake, had finally proposed marriage to her in a well-planned, choreographed event in Kansas City. Knowing what was happening with her mother that day, Karen was both excited and distraught.

Unbeknownst to her, both Shelley and I knew this news was coming, and pretty much to the precise date and moment. Back in August, Jake had visited our house to tell us he wanted to marry Karen, and that he planned to propose later in the year. Jake is a *great* guy, and we were pleased to welcome him to the family. Little did we know, then, that his popping the question would ultimately coincide with one of the most difficult times of our lives. It made for quite a bitter-sweet evening.

I was able to wake Shelley up for a few minutes so Karen could tell her, personally. They spoke for a short time and shared some tears that were simultaneously tinged with joy and sadness. Shelley then said softly, "I'm sorry, Honey, but I can't talk anymore. I'm exhausted, and I have to rest." I took the phone, Shelley closed her eyes and went right back to sleep.

Karen was still crying a little when I got back on the line. "Oh my God, it sounds terrible," she said. "Do you want me to come home right now?"

"It's been awful," I disclosed with a deep sigh. "But you're two hours away, and there's nothing you could do even if you were here. So just try to have a nice celebration tonight, because getting engaged is a big occasion."

"Ok, Dad. And I *will* be home on the 23rd for Christmas," she promised.

I was hoping Shelley could sleep through the remainder of the night, but a second wave of sickness hit a little after 10:00 pm. And it was every bit as ferocious as the first. Since it was afterhours, I frantically called the oncologist who was on late-night hospital duty, hoping there was something that could be done to calm the sickness. There really wasn't much he could say or do other than having her take another anti-nausea pill and pushing fluids if she could possibly keep them down. This was chemotherapy, after all. It was just the start of our new normal. Shelley vomited numerous times for another hour before things finally settled down.

I brought her back to the couch, put the blanket back on her, and she quickly returned to an almost coma-like sleep. I turned off the lights and lay down on the loveseat nearby so I could be right there the moment she needed me.

Shelley awoke at about 3:00 am, and I gave her another Compazine. She said she felt a *little* better and was able to keep this one down. After falling back asleep again, she woke up at 6:00. By that time, the nausea had clearly subsided, but her fatigue was enormous. She had no appetite whatsoever. She knew she needed to drink water or some electrolyte-infused liquids as much as she could in order to rehydrate from the vomiting spells. And eating something – anything – was also encouraged, if at all possible. She slowly ate half a piece of buttered toast and drank a small cup of water. It was all she could manage.

The rest of the day included a lot of extended naps, with a little food and drink in between. She was so weak she could only sit up for a few minutes at a time. That afternoon, Nick came home after his last final exam and was happy to spend some time with his mother. He, too, wanted to help care for her.

With the passage of each day, Shelley slowly regained her strength. By the time Christmas arrived, she was awake for much of the day, and she was strong enough to sit up for longer periods of time. She'd regained much of her appetite. She could carry on conversations. She could occasionally get up and walk to another room without my assistance. These were our little victories. We certainly didn't have the Christmas celebration we'd expected prior to diagnosis, but we made everything as traditional as we could. Karen and Nick were profoundly helpful in that capacity.

CHAPTER 4

Cancer vs. Christmas Magic

*The best of all gifts around any Christmas tree: the presence of
a happy family all wrapped up in each other.*

-Burton Hillis

The timing of a cancer diagnosis during the Christmas season can
test even the most indomitable of holiday spirits. But in spite of
the ominous cancer cloud hovering over our heads and the lingering chemo effects of Shelley's terrible December 21 treatment, we
hoped Christmas would still be enjoyable – well, relatively speaking
of course. It was nice to have Karen and Nick in Columbia to join us.
Shelley and I had decided in advance that we would do our best not
to let cancer completely take Christmas away from us. And though
we fell well short in a number of areas, we carried out as many of our
two-decades-long family traditions as best we could. Karen gleefully
pitched in as she, with some help from Nick, worked diligently during
the afternoon of Christmas Eve in making and decorating Christmas
cookies from old family recipes.

That first chemo treatment just physically sucked the life out of
Shelley for a few days, and I'll freely admit that the entire time since
the December 6 diagnosis had been an emotional struggle for me.
Because of the endless appointments and the treatment effects, we
weren't able to finish Christmas shopping, and the presents we got
for one another and the kids went pretty much unwrapped. We did

manage to get a few of them into gift bags, but most of the presents were simply left in their original store bags under the tree. We were also unable to make our traditional trek to a local, iconic downtown candy store for our yearly stocking stuffers. Sadly, and for the first time since Shelley and I were married, our Christmas stockings hung flat on the fireplace when we turned in on Christmas Eve, well before 10:00. We didn't have the strength or energy to do anything more.

Since our cancer nightmare began, I'd had great difficulty sleeping. Therefore, it came as no surprise that I lay in bed wide-awake at 3:30 am on Christmas morning. So I decided to go out to the living room and lie down on the couch. I thought that turning on the tree lights might provide a little relaxation. When I plugged them in, however, I was quite surprised to see, in the dim multicolored glow, that things around the tree and fireplace were not at all as we'd left them a few hours earlier.

I noticed that much of what previously was in shopping bags somehow got transferred to tagged gift bags or were wrapped in festive holiday paper. Furthermore, there were a number of additional packages under the tree, and all four of the once-flat stockings were stuffed to capacity. It was eerily similar to the Christmas-morning scenes we used to create for our kids when they were little and still believed in Jolly Old St. Nicholas. Holy crap, I thought, *did Santa really did make a midnight visit to our home?* Was this Christmas magic?

Obviously, these merry extras were a result of something even better – the heartfelt efforts of our own St. Nick and St. Karen. I later learned those two stayed up until well after 2:00 am, quietly and frantically working to make this difficult Christmas as magical as possible. If that didn't beat all. I grinned and shook my head in pleasant incredulity. I then turned on some Christmas music at very low volume and *finally* managed to drift back to sleep for a bit on the couch.

It was still dark when I woke up at about 6:00 am. For a little more holiday ambience to complement the tree lights and soft carols, I lit a log in the fireplace. For life necessity, I put on some freshly ground holiday blend coffee. It had snowed some the day before. And while the coffee was brewing, I peered through the kitchen window and saw that the white blanket still covered our lawn. The soft radiance of our outdoor Christmas lights illuminating through the snow on the bushes and outside stairway handrail was simply breathtaking. It was certainly looking a lot like Christmas.

No one else was up, yet, and as I took my first drink of piping hot coffee, I briefly had a moment of "other than that, how did you like the play, Mrs. Lincoln?" I sat and thought about how nice the anticipation of the day *would* have been were it not for this terrible hand that was dealt to my beautiful wife. Even as adults, Karen and Nick would have excitedly opened their presents. Shelley and I would have basked in the exhilaration of another successful holiday gift-giving operation. Throughout the afternoon, we would so much enjoy the kitchen's anticipatory aromas of preparing the grand Christmas dinner. And after a late dessert of homemade pumpkin pie and Christmas cookies, we'd conclude the evening sitting by the blazing fireplace and brightly lit tree, drinking toasts to one another while sipping fine wine and 18-year-old single-malt scotch as we capped off another glorious holiday season.

Sadly, I knew little of that would be happening today.

But then a sense of perspective entered the halls of my emotionally fragile mind. While we'd been consumed and devastated by our own crisis, cancer had most certainly not limited itself to the Hardeman family. I sat and thought about some of the faces of hopelessness I'd seen at Missouri Cancer Associates a couple of weeks before. I remembered that many other people were experiencing the same, terrible ordeal we were. And I considered the veritable tidal wave of support we had from friends. It was care that previously lay dormant until our chaos of diagnosis hit, which led many of those friends to quickly come to the aid of our cancer-stricken family. They brought us food and wonderful gifts. They spent time listening to us, even while we emotionally fell apart trying to cope. They gave rides and ran errands for us. They endlessly texted and emailed with me when I needed to vent, sometimes at 3:00 in the morning. Many of those dear friends had certainly gone *well* beyond any requisite call of duty they may have initially felt. I thought about the unrelenting, brilliant light of love that shines on us.

In spite of Karen's and Nick's late-night holiday labors, everyone was up by 8:00 am to open presents. Shelley was *finally* strong enough to sit up for longer than a few minutes at a time, and she, too, was able to enjoy a bit of good, hot coffee. Our kids then proceeded to take over the normal parenting duties in distributing gift bags and packages. They also handed us our stockings they'd filled with nuts and candy. I proudly sported the present from Nick I liked best, a bright pink "fight like a girl" breast-cancer-awareness T-shirt. In addition, he even had a special T-shirt made for me that perfectly blended my favorite basketball team's logo and "Relay For Life," the American Cancer Society fundraiser that Shelley and I participated in together for many years. Shelley put on her gift from me, a specially made gold and diamond pendant, which was inscribed, *With you every step of the way*. It turned out that, in spite of everything, we were able to enjoy Christmas morning.

Karen's fiancé, Jake, came over in the late afternoon and joined our celebration into the evening. Thanks to some grocery shopping Karen had done for us the day before, she and I managed to prepare a fairly decent Christmas dinner. Afterward, we all sat down to watch *The Polar Express*, which is Shelley's favorite holiday movie. By then, she was feeling much more like her old self.

It was, indeed, a pleasant and memorable Christmas. But, admittedly, that day I was already looking forward to future Christmases with Shelley, and hopefully without the cancer cloud hanging over us. To paraphrase a sentimental line from the TV show *Friends*, the love and support given to us by our own friends and family have made us feel like the luckiest people in the world. And, together, Shelley and I both want to spend the rest of our lives – the next 30 years or so – trying to make them all feel the same way.

Since Shelley had no desire to consume any alcohol, the five of us brought Christmas night to a close by lightly clinking champagne flutes of sparkling white grape juice. We made our toast to her.

And to her future good health.

And to our cherished, helpful friends.

And to St. Karen and St. Nick.

And … to Christmas magic.

CHAPTER 5

AC Rounds 2, 3, and 4 Were a Much Different Story

Don't let go
You've got the music in you
One dance left
This world is gonna pull through
Don't give up
You've got a reason to live
Can't forget
We only get what we give.
          -From "You Get What You Give" by The New Radicals

Though the medical community is sometimes unfairly rebuked for not having found cures for viruses that cause the common cold, I am astounded by how much cancer research has evolved since my father's illness in the late 1980s and early '90s. When those advancements were coupled with Shelley's physical ability to overcome some of the debilitating chemotherapy effects, her bounce-back was comparatively amazing.

By December 28 she said she felt "practically normal," when we had another medical appointment. This consultation included a very productive discussion with one of our oncology nurses who was determined to make adjustments to the antiemetic regimen for the next round. She seemed confident that Shelley's nausea could be significantly reduced for the impending January 4 treatment. We weren't so sure, though we obviously hoped that would be the case. The thought of repeating Shelley's previous reaction each time for three more Adriamycin/Cytoxan treatments was almost unbearable.

We drove to Missouri Cancer Associates on the morning of January 4 for Shelley's second round of AC accompanied by our ever-increasing apprehension. As we waited in the infusion room for Nurse Lindsay to begin the process again, good friend Mark texted me the iconic 1965 photo of Muhammad Ali (then, Cassius Clay) hovering over and screaming at a sprawled-on-the-canvas Sonny Liston with the obvious symbolism of Shelley beating up on her cancer. When I showed it to her, she smiled nervously and said, "Let's hope."

Since it took place earlier in the morning than the previous infusion, we didn't have lunch during this treatment as we had done the preceding round. With vivid memories of violent nausea entrenched firmly in our minds, we were even more uneasy regarding this outcome. But during the two-week hiatus prior to the second treatment, I did read that the first is often the worst of the chemo for short-term reaction. (Of course, I'm not referring to the nasty, cumulative side effects that build over a span of weeks and months.)

Much to our delight, round two of Shelley's chemotherapy came and went, and with a vastly different outcome from the previous infusion. Whereas the afternoon and evening of that first treatment resulted in severe nausea, vomiting, and extended periods of very deep sleep, this time it was far easier on the sickness front. *Far* easier. It almost seemed too easy. And we both loved every second of it. Though there is no question that she still felt physically bulldozed, which necessitated equally long naps, her appetite this time around was almost completely normal. We could only hope that the next two sessions of this intense AC treatment would have similar results. The new nausea drug procedure appeared to have worked. Things have really changed on that front since my father went through his chemotherapy three decades earlier. Of course, most importantly, we hoped these treatments would do precisely what they were put into her body to do. That would remain to be seen, as we still had the vast majority of this rough journey to travel.

On occasion, Shelley even felt up to having a few visitors, although January usually means cold and flu season is in full swing. With strong chemotherapy throughout her body, her immune system was compromised in spite of her injected white-blood-cell-promoting drugs. Obviously, we had to be hypersensitive in avoiding any kind of infection. [Think necessity of social distancing and home lockdowns during the 2020 COVID-19 pandemic, but on a much smaller scale.] With cancer fighting, there's no such thing as "just a cold." Which meant that I more than willingly played the role of germ defense gatekeeper, protecting Shelley from those with any type of prospective illness.

I had no problem with the idea of turning away visitors who might insist their cough or sniffles were "probably nothing." Or those who inexplicably dissed the entire medical community's scientifically sound, safe, and collective admonitions by refusing to get a flu vaccine. And that is because I remember well the several times when my father became ill with various viral maladies during his chemo treatments. Each bout took him weeks from which to fully recover, and, worse, it sometimes delayed his needed treatment as a result. I must confess, therefore, that all of Shelley's visitors were closely scrutinized with what must have occasionally seemed like third-degree interrogation prior to their admission into our house.

We were also concerned about the prospect of illness surrounding Shelley when she was able to go in to work. Thankfully, co-workers Sherry and Crystal took it upon themselves to completely disinfect the cubicles, printers, keyboards, and anything else Shelley might touch around her work area, and, bless them both, they did so *every single morning* prior to her arrival.

As stated, Shelley's second treatment brought on as much fatigue, but with far less nausea. Her chemo, however, took its toll in other ways. We knew the day was coming when her hair would begin to fall out. She also knew she wouldn't be feeling good about it. Just two treatments in, she had quite a bit of hair loss during showers and morning hair preparation. She decided on January 9 that it was time to get the clippers and cut it off. I did the deed, and I knew what it was doing to her self-esteem. Nick was present during the process, and he was visibly affected, emotionally, when he saw his mother without any hair. But in the bigger picture, she had already obtained a wig at the end of December, and it looked great. More importantly, she felt better about herself while wearing it.

The new normal part of the every-two-weeks AC treatment was that it took a full week for Shelley to recover before she went back to work for a week. And then the process started over again. And, of course, she had to return to work when possible since her health insurance was tied to her employment. Her professional obligations clearly took a physical toll on her. She would get home by 5:30 pm and be asleep on the couch well before 8:00.

At this point, we had two remaining AC treatments to go before the 12 rounds of Taxol would commence in February.

Round 3 on January 18: "It's softer!"

Amid the calamity-of-cancer narrative throughout my CaringBridge posts, I always discussed any small victories we had on which to rest a few hopes. Sometimes that meant something as minor as having appointments go as planned, time-wise. It was also as big as maintaining her appetite without the nausea after chemo. And on the morning of January 18, we got another small victory.

Before the start of that day's chemo treatment, we met with Dr.

Makarian. When she felt the tumor area two weeks prior, she had said there was no change. However, when she felt it the morning of the treatment, she said, in a *very* pleased tone of voice, "It's softer!" While, obviously, there were no guarantees at that point, a tumor getting softer suggests it may be losing its mass due to the chemo killing off some of the cancer cells. It certainly gave us more reason to hope. And as the saying goes, there's no place like hope, right?

Since Shelley's antiemetic regimen change was so successful the previous session, we said to our nurse, "Whatever you did the last time, please do it exactly the same way." We stood ready with oral anti-nausea meds but hoped that we'd have a repeat performance from January 4. Which is precisely what we got. When we arrived home from that third AC chemotherapy at lunchtime, Shelley almost ravenously ate a meal of two large chicken legs, a glass of milk, and a carton of yogurt. And, again, we had no nausea!

Each time we finished a round of treatment, we put up a very small sign on our dining room door railing that said, "one more chemo down." At that point, we had three up with 13 to go.

Completion of round 4: our first true milestone

After the fourth infusion on February 1, we returned home at about 1:30 pm, and we were pleased. For the third consecutive treatment, Shelley experienced no nausea. And on this day, we reached a significant milestone. Though we were only a quarter of the way through the 16 scheduled rounds (not to mention we had surgery and radiation to follow down the road as the year continued), it marked the completion of Shelley's final powerful, but dreaded, AC cocktail. It was a huge hurdle that this incredibly strong and resilient woman cleared. She had come such a long way from her initial, debilitating December 21 infusion.

But there was no question her treatment was revealing its cumulative effect. Though nausea, again, was thankfully not a factor in the equation, the fourth round definitely created the most fatigue. Typically, Shelley's energy level returned to normal within six or seven days, which allowed her to go into work afterward. This time around it was a good nine days before she had the strength to even think about returning to work.

Our oncologist was outwardly encouraged with the overall progress, however. She said that Shelley's tumor was even softer than two weeks before. Even more significant, Dr. Makarian said she actually had to search a bit to find it.

Following these four rounds of AC would be Taxol. And the regimen would change from infusions every two weeks to 12 weekly treatments, starting on February 16. Generally speaking (and, again, I am *not* a medical professional), the AC kills cancer cells by working to destroy their cellular DNA. This creates interference with recurrent division and reproduction, causing the cells to die.[17] Taxol also works to slow and stop cell division. We were told that while Taxol was supposed to be a little less intense and, thereby, more tolerable than the AC, it certainly could present undesirable side effects. Hand and foot neuropathy, muscle tightness, allergic reactions, skin problems, bone pain, fatigue, and irregular heartbeat could occur, according to Dr. Makarian. She also said that hair loss (which was moot, since Shelley had already lost all her hair) and nausea were experienced by some, but to a lesser degree.

This brought forth one of the great fallacies of cancer treatment. When some of our friends and family heard that this new therapy would be less severe than the previous, they often assumed all would be fine from that point on. And many of them even outwardly downplayed the new, upcoming side-effects. Since Shelley had weathered the AC storm, some friends rationalized that the rest should be comparatively easy.

But a change in treatment means a change in bodily reaction to the new chemicals. Less severe side effects to a new treatment can still be quite difficult to manage. Think of it this way: while a copperhead's snake venom kills far fewer people and is certainly less toxic than that of a rattlesnake, *who actually wants to be bitten by a copperhead?* There was no question Shelley and I were happy about the conclusion of AC. But as horrible as it was, at least it was predictable. And with new chemotherapy, there was the unsettling feeling of the unknown. How would she react to it? What would the next new normal be like?

Nonetheless, there was room for guarded optimism. This was another little victory we could celebrate. In our boxing analogies, Clay continued to repeatedly hit Liston. Rocky Balboa persisted in pummeling Clubber Lang. And Shelley never let up as she fought on in these epic battles.

CHAPTER 6

With Her Every Step of the Way

The true mark of maturity is when somebody hurts you, and you try to understand their situation instead of trying to hurt them back.

-Ryron Gracie

Short of having the condition, I can never *fully* empathize with, understand, or appreciate the punishing road a cancer fighter takes. I did experience a life-threatening situation involving coronary artery disease in late 2015. But it was essentially corrected through a 30-minute catheter procedure involving the insertion of stents to open two almost completely blocked branches of my right coronary artery. I was, according to my cardiologist, days from a fatal heart attack when I entered the hospital. But while I was literally dying one minute, I was fine the next at the conclusion of the procedure. I had a few months of cardiac-rehabilitation thereafter, but it was really nothing outside of my previously existing, normal exercise routine. In addition, I'll likely need to be on certain medications with relatively few side effects for the rest of my life. No harm no foul, from my perspective.

There's no half-hour fix for cancer, however. If someone is fortunate enough to have caught it in its earliest of stages, the malignancy sometimes can be surgically removed. This increases the chances of rendering the patient cancer-free, and, in the most fortuitous (and fortunate) of situations, without the necessity of any further treatment. But this isn't exactly the norm.

Cancer is often asymptomatic until there is considerable progression. This is why age- and gender-appropriate early detection measures such as colonoscopies, mammograms, prostate-specific antigen blood tests, pap smears, and a full-body skin check by a dermatologist are vitally important. They can potentially identify cancer in those early, much more treatable stages.

Otherwise, metastasis can go unnoticed for quite some time. And since much of the ensuing war is on the microscopic level, there may be no concluding litmus test, other than the passage of time, to see if the disease has truly been eradicated. Therefore, treatment might need to occur over an extended period and may take months, if not years. I watched what both my father and my wife underwent in their respective cancer treatments. I saw that not only were there extreme difficulties with each round, the cumulative effects continued to accrue. And various adjuvant medications that are taken for years after an extended chemo/surgery/radiation regimen may bring forth additional long-lasting side effects as well.

As fate would have it, my mother and I were exactly the same age when our spouses were diagnosed. We learned on September 6, 1985, that my father had stage IV non-Hodgkin's lymphoma. His disease was inoperable, as it had spread throughout his body. There would never be a cure for him. But his cancer *was* treatable, depending, of course, on how both he and the cancer responded to chemotherapy. His initial survival prognosis was estimated at anywhere from six months to 10 years. His venue of treatment was the renowned City of Hope National Medical Center in Duarte, California, which was a 40-mile, one-way commute for my parents in the heart of Southern California freeway traffic.

Dad lived for six years, four months, and three days before passing away. In that time, he endured the most horrible of chemo reactions, but he never complained. During a treatment hiatus, he was able to travel the world with my mother. He got some much needed summer R&R at our cabin in Utah. He attended my wedding in Iowa and saw, after witnessing a goodly number of my relationship disasters, that I had truly found my soulmate in Shelley. As a retired history professor, he continued his academic love for researching and writing. He did what we all should be doing *without* a cancer diagnosis: Each day he wasted no time and lived life to its fullest. Until he no longer could.

Both my parents were ferociously intelligent, articulate, and highly educated individuals. My father was a multi-award-winning professor at California State University, Long Beach with a Ph.D. from the University of California-Berkeley. My mother earned her master's degree in social ecology at the University of California-Irvine.

Mom sometimes exhibited Type A personality characteristics and occasionally, like many of us, had difficulty coping when faced with concurrent high-stress situations. It didn't help that her academic-programming job at UCI was demanding and pressure packed. Regardless, she was a consummate caregiver. But a stroke in 1988 manifestly slowed her vocal rate and decision-making processes. In retrospect, I think it may have actually made her even more thoughtful and reflective in her caregiving role. This was something I definitely noticed. Before *and* after her stroke, she cared for my father with grace and compassion during the last years of his life.

As one of their two adult sons, I was, back then, employed as an instructor at the University of Northern Iowa, which meant that I lived nearly 1800 miles from my parents. Therefore, I played no part in caregiving for 10-11 months out of the year. When I'd visit for several weeks during winter and summer breaks, I'd accompany them to chemo treatments and run errands for them as needed. But it was only on a temporary basis as, eventually, I had to return to my job in Iowa.

While it was definitely stressful, caregiving never seemed to elude my mother's ordinary actions. It was just what she did. I now know that I didn't fully appreciate what those six-plus years were doing to her, physically and emotionally. Dad passed away when they were both only 68, but Mom lived another 24 years. She never remarried. She didn't even date. She never got over losing the love of her life, her husband of more than 45 years. She died two years before Shelley's diagnosis.

Cancer fighting and caregiving: the ultimate team sport

Caregiving is most certainly not on the level of having cancer. Nonetheless, I found that coping with the extensive obligations, un-certainties, and apprehensions could be incredibly hectic. As a result, I know that my friends and family worried about me almost as much as about Shelley during this time of tumult and turmoil. Caregivers must find their own pathways and strength to keep going through-out the cancer ordeal. The role repeatedly tested my emotional and physical limits. Nonetheless, positive caregiving as a spouse can be quite important. Recent studies suggest that a productive significant-other relationship is medically beneficial in creating a good outcome for breast cancer patients.[18]

To be successful, one has to have the right caregiving frame of mind. As difficult as it was to carry out all the responsibilities, for me it meant unhesitatingly putting Shelley's needs above *all else in life*, regardless of what I was asked to do. With a cancer diagnosis came a rapid makeover in life-issue priorities. All other problems immediate-ly paled in comparison. Prior to Shelley's cancer, I was, like my moth-er, often bogged down in work issues that seemed crucial at the time. I would lose sleep over situations involving unhappy administrators and students. In addition, I was an avid sports fan. I seemingly lived and died with the outcomes of my favorite college and professional teams. I yelled and screamed when watching them on television and shrieked in euphoria when they won, almost as if the consequence of their loss or victory equated some profound life event.

But on diagnosis day, that all came to an abrupt halt. At that moment I saw just how much my current life-drama issues were not only trivial by comparison, they almost seemed contrived. So I quickly adopted some survival changes: Short of online teaching obligations, I no longer bring my grading or administrative work home to do. I've also learned to psychologically leave at campus whatever professional issues that might interfere with home duties. Since then, I note that I don't always get administrative work completed by the time administrators want it done. More often than not, they've been very understanding. Also, while I still watch sports on television occasionally, it's not nearly as often as I once did. I simply no longer care about the outcomes. Since Shelley's diagnosis took place, only one thing in life has mattered to me.

Just like many successful couples when they start out, Shelley and I had no sense about any future together when, back in 1988, our paths unexpectedly and serendipitously crossed. Prior to then, we'd both suffered through our shares of unhealthy past romantic relationships.

But, together, we immediately clicked. Her personality was infectiously positive. Whenever I spoke with her, she treated me as if our conversation was the pinnacle of her day. It soon turned out that we were looking for precisely what the other willingly offered: uncompromising love, devotion, honesty, openness, respect, equality, trust, empathy, and commitment. Her entrance into my world was the very best of life-changing events. From the start, we truly enjoyed one another's company, and that has only developed and intensified over the decades. We talk. We listen. We laugh at ourselves, even in confident self-deprecation. We praise one another. We agree on most things in life and disagree with the utmost of mutual respect. We support one another at all times.

With each interaction and every shared gaze, we synergistically bring out the best in the other. We recognize that not knocking someone down isn't the same as helping them up, and we *always* extend a hand to help each other up when needed. The manner in which she treats me makes me aspire to be a better husband. We are, indeed, a *team*.

But when cancer entered our lives, we were confined to playing overlapping, but different, positions in a new game, with the hope of not impeding the other. Shelley was the only player on our team to *experience* treatment. The nausea. The pain. The hair loss. The neuropathy. The fatigue. The surgery recovery. The needles. Relatively few people outside of cancer fighters truly know these realities. Prolonged cancer treatment is one of the most trying and difficult medical paths any human being could take. And I was the caregiver who couldn't alleviate any of her physical discomfort. I could only watch what was happening.

Imagine having a front-row seat at a major league baseball game (or any sporting event). Because of the close proximity, you are positioned with a far better vantage point than most others at the stadium in experiencing all the sights and sounds of the game. You see the true speed of a pitch and the quickness of infielders turning a double play. You hear the plate umpire bellowing out balls and strikes, the pop from a throw hitting a player's glove or mitt, the solid crack of the bat on a home run swing, and a player's agonizing scream of pain after a serious knee injury. You may vividly imagine, but you don't actually *feel* a blazing 98 mph fastball hitting your ribs. You won't suffer the concussive force of a violent collision between two speedy, athletic outfielders in a dead sprint chasing down the same fly ball. You don't experience your thigh being pierced by the cleats of a baserunner sliding hard into second base. And that is because you're not *in* the game; you're only a spectator.

But now envision that one of the players is your parent, son, daughter, or significant other. Your lives are intertwined outside of the game, and you therefore have a personally vested interest in that player's well-being. You care about him/her as much as (or more than) anyone else. If your player gets hurt, you don't feel the bodily damage and are not directly subjected to any of the recovery or rehabilitation. But you're still expressly affected by your loved one's injury more than any other fan. It's because of your distinctive relationship with the player. Few, if any, could feel your emotional pain, because they don't have that close connection.

This is what it's like to be a cancer caregiver for your spouse or other immediate family member. I didn't experience the cancer and treatment, but I had a front-row seat, which was the next best – or worst – perspective. As a result, the psychological pain is probably on par with that of the patient. I watched all the suffering close up, so my position in this game was as a direct participant on the recovery team.

In turn, Shelley's cancer-fighting perception of my caregiving was limited to being a recipient of and witness to how I carried out my duties. She could certainly comment about it (and she sometimes did), but she couldn't feel my psychological pain or my own mounting fatigue. She could only observe my nonverbal expressions. She wasn't the one who was temporarily charged with working full-time while doing all the domestic work and providing the caregiving. In my role, I sometimes found this comparable to juggling three full-time jobs. While I could never tell her how to cope with her cancer and treatment, she couldn't tell me how to manage, either, because she wasn't playing *my* position. Since we both had to do our parts for her successful recovery, dual empathy was critical.

Obviously, Shelley's diagnosis was an exceptionally frightening time. The initial prospect of losing her was unbearable. And there's no question that, in return for the help I tried to constantly provide, she simultaneously did the same in offering her emotional support for her sometimes overwhelmed husband. For example, she was well aware of my personal need to be with her at her appointments. And I was grateful that she purposely scheduled them on days and times when I could join her in spite of how it may have affected her own professional duties.

One of the many communication courses I teach is college public speaking, which is, according to numerous and repeated studies, the greatest fear among Americans. Therefore, because of my profession, I've had countless opportunities to observe how that emotion affects my students. Fear does different things to people. Some members of my classes are patently immobilized by stage fright. With all the sets of audience eyes focused upon them, their energy is depleted, their voices are soft and monotone, and they won't establish any semblance of eye contact with their audience. They are utterly paralyzed in fear. This is what speech scholars refer to as *debilitative stage fright*. Some students' fears are so pronounced that they can even preclude any progress in public speaking because they are limited by self-fulfilling prophecy. Since they firmly believe they will fail in spite of preparation level, they often won't spend any time and energy preparing at all. And this only intensifies their fears for the following speech.

On the other hand, other students are somehow able to harness their fears to sustain maximum preparation, prompting continuous rehearsal beyond their professor's expectations, which usually facilitates a more productive outcome. As a result, they raise their performance level higher than they ever anticipated.

This is how I tried to see myself as a caregiver for Shelley. If I have been successful in this role, it was due, in large part, to my own fear of the disease's conceivable terminal outcome. Aside from the love I feel for her, fear, more than anything else, drove me to stay at her side with every appointment, treatment, and day of home care.

I was a bit surprised by the occasions when oncology staff commented positively on my repeated presence during Shelley's appointments during the beginning phases of test and other consultations. We certainly noticed that some patients were accompanied by caregivers while others were not. Since I assumed most other spouses would do the same, those compliments caught me a bit off guard. As a result, I usually I deflected them by saying, "I need to be here for my own well-being, and she'd do the same thing if the situation were reversed." A Swedish proverb describes our marriage perfectly: "Shared joy is a double joy, shared sorrow is half a sorrow."[19] As consummate team members, Shelley and I always have each other's backs. When one of us is down, the other offers unadulterated support. On the other hand, we celebrate any individual successes together, because we know that a better player makes for a better team.

While a cancer diagnosis is terrible regardless of significant-other status, I cannot imagine how much more difficult it must be to face alone. Sadly, our surgeon and oncologist mentioned of some of their breast cancer patients whose husbands withdrew completely. A few, they said, let their wives attend every appointment and treatment alone. That is inconceivable to me. Prior to COVID-19 in 2020 when clinic policy disallowed me from accompanying her, there were but two appointments when I thought it best to stay home because of my own illness. "Where is Keith?" was the exclamatory question asked of Shelley not only by the receptionist, but also the nurses and oncologist. Clearly, they, too, saw us as a team.

And then there were our employers who also served us well in the capacity of extended team members. As a college professor, I am quite fortunate to be in a vocation that possesses some inherent scheduling flexibility. Since the timing of Shelley's diagnosis came at the end of an academic term, I had about four weeks before classes would begin for the following semester. Therefore, I could easily dedicate the entirety of my time and energy toward emotional and physical caregiving while the cancer ordeal began to take shape.

When the new semester commenced, I was able to do some of

my job from home or from the cancer clinic during Shelley's appointments and treatments. By way of smartphone, computer, and tablet, I could provide teaching lessons online, when necessary. I emailed with students who needed individual help. Video or speakerphone calls could let me "attend" committee meetings.

Obviously, we all have professional responsibilities that must be met, even in the worst of times. The key for Shelley and me was working with our supervisors and coworkers to find measures that allowed us to meet both professional and medical obligations. As a healthy, longtime employee, Shelley had accrued sick time and was able to use it throughout her treatment. But we both kept open the lines of communication with our employers and relevant colleagues by constantly updating them. As a result, the compassion they exhibited was often unparalleled. They kindly gave us the professional space we sometimes required. "Tell us what you need," was their constant, underlying message. They made it clear to us that we were not alone in this battle. I suspect people in most organizations react similarly (and shame on the ones who don't). I quickly discovered that it was very good to have the extended team of my college president, deans, faculty and staff peers, and students in my corner.

If I were truly going to help my wife fight cancer, there were harsh interpersonal realities with which we needed to come to terms. Shelley and I knew that her cancer was something that could ultimately kill her. Or it could be a chronic disease she must doggedly fight over the course of many years. She may end up beating it, altogether. But regardless, it was going to be a long, exhaustive, and painful journey. I wouldn't be helpful to her if we were bickering over inane issues, which would only make life more difficult for her. There could be no productive outcome if I ever implicitly communicated the senseless idea that being married to a cancer fighter was somehow more difficult than *being* a cancer fighter. I wanted her to reserve all her strength and energy for battling cancer. Whatever I did as a caregiver, my goal was always to put the team above myself and to be certain not to make a bad situation worse in how I handled my responsibilities. Therefore, it was imperative that I should *never* tackle my teammate. Though I'm certain I inadvertently fell short on this front several times, I tried to do my very best.

During my teaching units in interpersonal conflict resolution, I initially ask my students what their ultimate goal is when engaging with someone in an argument or dispute. Their collective answers are almost always unanimously the same: to win. Unfortunately, the win/lose paradigm all but insures that the problem being addressed will not be resolved to both parties' satisfaction. Additionally, that approach also means overlooking the differences between battles and wars. While the content of some arguments can be critical, many issues are just not that important. But they're still sometimes carried out to a destructive, win-at-all-cost finish. Though I've sometimes been guilty of this in the past, I've learned over the years that some things just aren't worth fighting over.

All marriages have occasions of disagreement, but when cancer is involved, it's a proverbial game changer. I kept the big picture in the forefront of my mind. Whenever we had a minor dispute, I did my best to keep my ego in check. There are far more important things in life than a self-indulgent "need" to win a trivial argument with someone who's battling a life-threatening illness. Shelley was already fighting cancer. Therefore, I didn't want her to squander energy fighting me too. Again, in order for the goal of survival to be met, I felt her needs should come first. *Always*. Allowing her to make decisions she momentarily felt strongly about did not lessen my manhood. As President John F. Kennedy said at his 1961 inaugural speech, "...civility is not a sign of weakness."[20] In this case, neither was any of my caregiving acquiescence.

Nevertheless, cancer treatment itself can affect a host of potential issues that increase chances of interpersonal conflict. As I explained earlier, chemotherapy brings with it an abundance of nasty side effects. One that I haven't yet mentioned is what many cancer patients call *chemo brain*. The American Cancer Society describes it as a very real "mental fog" that affects one's thought processes in a variety of ways.[21] It differs from patient to patient. Some feel it only in the short term. Others have more intense, long-term experiences.

As her chemotherapy began, Shelley confessed early on that she was having occasional memory glitches with things she previously had no problem recalling. She couldn't multitask as well. She sometimes forgot names and places. And, intermittently, there were times when her irritation fuse was a little shorter with me. As a logical, well-educated, intelligent, and clear-thinking individual, she experienced great frustration with this condition.

Shelley's bright, upbeat personality never changed with chemo. But I noticed her sporadically snapping at me over what I sometimes thought were insignificant issues. In nearly three decades of gratifying, pre-cancer marriage, our arguments had been relatively few. However, like most couples, even we occasionally quarreled over the silliest things that only seemed important in the heat of the moment. But during her cancer treatment, I felt it would be best to do whatever possible to stay focused on the big picture and de-escalate any potential hostilities. Therefore, if she criticized me during this time, my set response was something to the effect of a calm, "You're right, Honey, I'm really sorry" rather than getting defensive. And prospective arguments never materialized as a result. Canadian cartoonist Lynn Johnston appropriately refers to apologies as "the superglue of life."[22]

Now if you're reading this and saying to yourself, *I don't know why Keith would apologize if he's not wrong*, you're missing the point. Generally speaking, my apologies usually mean one of two things: 1) I'm adult enough to admit when I'm actually wrong, or 2) I'm smart enough to realize that a good relationship should be more important than my ego, even if I may not be wrong. This was clearly not the time for me to take things personally. I'm not advocating an apology in response to every situation when someone is immaturely throwing a tantrum. What I *am* saying is that *there should be no marital-issue scorekeeping when cancer is involved.*[23]

When my cancer-fighting partner picked at me about something I saw as trivial, I tried to just give her a free pass without getting defensive. It was certainly possible that some of her comments were motivated more by chemo brain (or just feeling perpetually lousy) than anything else. Because of a conceivable spiral effect, verbally hitting back may be like lighting a metaphorical match in a fireworks stand. Instead, I wanted to use cooperation over competition. I think Shelley noticed and appreciated me for it in the long run. When she was happy, *I* was happy. And in the words of jazz artist Michael Franks, "I'd rather be happy than right."[24]

There is another fine interpersonal line that cancer caregivers quickly need to identify. This is far easier said than done, because it will be in constant flux. The line? Being able to figure out and negotiate what cancer fighters can and cannot do for themselves while coping with treatment that limits their physical abilities versus what they need to be able to do to maintain a sense of independence and "self-normalcy." It may take a lot of trial and error to determine (and reestablish) where those boundaries are.

Shelley has always been a very strong and independent person. Not woman. *Person.* She is stronger than most people I know (including me, as I watched her handling her cancer with grace and maturity), regardless of gender. Even during the worst of treatment, she hated relying on other people to do things she wanted to do herself. Or at least those things she'd always been able to do in the past. She takes exception to being patronized, and she doesn't want to be seen as not fulfilling what she views as her obligations. Mostly, she's refused to let others define her personhood by her cancer.

"I can do it" was Shelley's occasionally defiant mantra when I sometimes offered to do things for her during treatment. Perhaps it was because she assumed she could do something but then, with self-disappointment and frustration, learned that she couldn't. There were times she wasn't sure, but she wanted to try for the sake of trying. Or it might have been that she truly felt well enough to do things that she once did and wished to resume doing. I wouldn't know until I watched how everything played itself out. But often – for better or, sometimes, worse – I would simply intervene.

At the start of the intense chemotherapy that knocked Shelley out for several days at a time, I temporarily took over virtually all household duties that we'd previously shared – the cooking, the dishes, cleaning, laundry, snow shoveling, et al. Especially during the first six weeks when she was physically incapable much of the time. I didn't do the work perfectly, and I was often late in completing various tasks. And I will say that none of my chores were lost on Shelley, as I think she may have been simultaneously appreciative while almost jealously resentful. She went to work the days she could, but she needed to stay in bed, resting, on others. There were weeks when she could only work half days, and she sometimes got a little stir-crazy. Quick, on-setting fatigue replaced the energy of this once dynamic, vibrant woman. Since I was doing housework in addition to my full-time job, I wondered if she began to feel guilty. She told me, in no uncertain terms, to stop trying to do everything myself. I, on the other hand, assured her (and, perhaps, bullheadedly so) that I in fact *could* manage it all. Sometimes that meant staying up until midnight or rising at 4:00 am – or both – as I tried to keep up.

Late one evening when I began doing the dishes, Shelley came into the kitchen and picked up a dishtowel to dry them. I should have said nothing – I *really* should have said *nothing* – but instead I told her I didn't need or want her help and that she should sit down and rest in the living room. And that's when we finally had our one and only legitimate argument about patient/caregiving roles. It lasted literally 30 seconds.

"Stop treating me like a cancer patient!" she demanded, and not softly.

"But you *are* a cancer patient!" I countered in nearly equal volume.

"That doesn't mean you get to decide what I can or can't do!"

"I know! But you can't treat me like I have no role, here! You have to work with me in figuring this out, to do what's best for you to get through this!"

Sadly, we were both saying the same thing: We desperately wanted the old Shelley back. I still insisted that she leave the kitchen so I could finish doing the dishes myself. She very reluctantly complied. Since it was about bedtime, I left the clean dishes on the counter to air dry. "Just leave them there," I instructed her afterward, "and I'll put them away tomorrow after I get home from work." She agreed. At least for the moment.

The next day, Shelley returned home before I did. When I arrived, I saw that the dishes had been put away, and she sheepishly apologized for raising her voice the night before. "I'm sorry for yelling last night," she said. "I know you were doing what you thought was best. And you were right. I have to accept that even though I want to do them, there are a lot of things I can't do, right now."

"No worries, Honey," I replied. "It was my fault, anyway. I shouldn't have told you not to help." Then she confessed that her moment of realization occurred an hour before I got home. In the process of putting dishes into the cupboard, she dropped a ceramic coffee mug. Sentimentally, it was her favorite cup, a gift to her from our daughter. It upset Shelley as she helplessly watched it fall to the floor and shatter. The pain and neuropathy in her hands from chemotherapy just didn't allow her to properly grip it. Though it was a bit of an emotional and frustrating setback for her, the good part was that she finally realized her physical limitations, and it led to a very open and frank discussion about our respective roles and fluid boundaries.

As the caregiver, I needed to recognize Shelley's priority to do whatever she could on the physical front. While it wasn't my objective to deny her of any confidence-building activity that helping around the house might provide, I wanted her to feel assured that I harbored no resentment about doing the extra work. I was willing to do it all, and for as long as it took for her to completely recover. She said she'd be honest with herself and not hesitate to ask me for help when she felt she might need it. She also promised not to feel patronized if I offered a comment such as, "Let me do that for you."

For my part, I agreed to stop being an overbearing "helicopter caregiver," hovering over her every move (which I probably had been, more often than not). It was a very productive discussion. Since then, we've succeeded in calmly respecting, adhering to, and (re)negotiating those boundaries.

Self-image, attraction, intimacy, and cancer

If anyone is wondering if there still can be romance after a cancer diagnosis, my answer, in the short run, is an unhesitating *yes!* But there's a little more to the story.

Whether it's chemotherapy, radiation, surgery recovery, or other medications, there's very little in the treatment routine that makes a cancer-fighter feel good, physically or emotionally. Patients undergoing chemo will, more than likely, lose much, or all, of their hair. This isn't limited to the scalp area. It also includes eyebrows, eyelashes, and pubic hair. ("At least I won't have to shave my legs," Shelley said, in lighthearted resignation.)

Less than a week after Shelley's second chemo treatment, her hair loss was so abundant that she asked me to cut off her remaining locks. As I removed what was left with the electric clippers, her emerging tears showed me how deeply it was affecting her. In response, both our adult children and I seriously and resolutely offered to shave our heads in solidarity. Shelley actually laughed out loud and said, "I appreciate the gesture, but *please* don't do it. If I don't want to see myself bald, why would I want to see my kids and husband bald when they don't have to be?" And that was the first time Shelley was able to bring a small bit of humor into the cancer equation. I immediately joined in.

"Oh, c'mon," I said, chuckling in return. I then referenced a *Seinfeld* episode we'd recently seen and asked, "Don't you want to act like George Costanza, look at me, and say, 'He's BAAALD'"? Shelley outwardly giggled, which, I thought, was a good sign. Since we knew the hair loss was coming, she was fitted for and purchased a wig couple of weeks beforehand. I posted a picture on CaringBridge of her wearing it, and it garnered a lot of positive feedback. Included were written comments from several of my male friends (who also were involuntarily without hair) chiming in with bald jokes and indicating that, unlike her, their hair loss was permanent. There also were many heartfelt compliments about how good she looked in her new wig. All of it really seemed to lift her spirits in helping her acceptance of the situation.

Predictably, Shelley's hair loss initially had a strong emotional impact on her. She dealt with it, in part, by wearing her wig at work and in other public places. When she'd come home, she replaced it with a thin stocking cap. After losing her hair, she never allowed any photographs of herself without something covering the top of her head. She was also very clear in communicating its effect on her self-image – she did not feel attractive. And this could have negatively affected her perception of marital relations at the outset. Not to mention that when she already felt worn out and crappy most of the time, intimacy, understandably, wasn't often at the forefront of her mind. If this is how your cancer-fighting spouse feels, *you have to accept and respect it*. When this happens in a cancer story, it can be a difficult paradox for the spousal caregiver to manage.

Hair or no hair, I felt it was important for Shelley to understand that I never lost any of my physical attraction to her, regardless of how her side effects manifested themselves. While I know she usually appreciated my flattery, she admitted she sometimes thought I was saying it out of obligation and pity. This was a double-bind message. If you compliment your cancer-fighting wife when she doesn't feel good about herself, she may think you're only saying things to make her feel better. But, of course, if you say nothing positive at all, she could interpret that as a strong nonverbal signal that you, indeed, have lost your attraction to her.

But what I needed to remember was that she was also thinking about how others would react to her ever-changing looks. If she didn't feel pretty, nothing I could say would convince her otherwise. Simply telling her, "You're still beautiful," does not show requisite empathy. If I focus my responses only on how *I* see her, I'm not acknowledging her anxieties about how others will, and she may feel invalidated because I'm not really hearing her.

I figured this out quickly when Shelley began talking about her looks in a self-deprecating manner. "Don't worry, you'll always be beautiful to me," I said, thinking that's what she wanted to hear. It wasn't. I soon realized she heard it as a counterproductive attempt to shut down her negative feelings. She shot back with a calm, but somewhat terse, "Darling, believe me that I'm grateful to have your support. But that's not my point, and you know it." She was right. I'm sure I must have sounded hopelessly patronizing.

What did work for me was communicating openly and honestly about my unconditional love while trying to outwardly empathize with and acknowledge the insecurities Shelley was naturally feeling. I remember a short conversation we had one morning while she was getting ready for work.

"I don't have any eyelashes to put mascara on," she said with deep frustration while looking at her reflection in the bathroom mirror. "And if I draw eyebrows, it might look stupid, and people could think I don't care about how I present myself."

I could have downplayed her concern with a dismissive, "No, they won't, it'll be fine," but I thought better of it. Instead, I said, "Yeah, they might," to validate her apprehension. "And, if any of them are so shallow as to say something about it," I continued, "just smile, look 'em straight in the eye and tell 'em 'I wish you better luck if *you* ever have to fight cancer.'"

Still gazing in the mirror, she pursed her lips, then grinned and nodded in the affirmative. "Yeah, you're right," she said. "It'll be OK. Thanks for the confidence boost." All she needed was for me to reaffirm her understandable anxieties. She came to her own positive conclusion without my committing the cardinal sin of telling her how she should be feeling.

I didn't really have much difficulty convincing Shelley that I was still passionately in love with her, emotionally *and* physically. However, I saw another prospective paradox in the realm of affection. While I was clear that I still found her to be desirable, I certainly hoped she wouldn't feel obligated to engage in intimacy if she felt miserable. Most importantly, I didn't want to do anything that might cause her some sort of physical harm.

There's a lot of great information about sex and cancer that's easily found on various legitimate cancer websites. But, awkward as we felt about it at the outset, we chose to have candid conversations with a member of our oncology team. We got straight, comfortable, nonjudgmental answers from one of our veteran nurses who addressed the issue with maximum professionalism: "Sex during cancer treatment is not only fine, we recommend it if Shelley's feeling up to it," was one thing the nurse told us. Suffice to say, when Shelley felt well, we were able to maintain a fairly normal romantic life throughout her treatments. But I always gave her space when she was the least bit hesitant.

Caregiving and burnout

Let me be very candid in saying that caregivers have to be aware of burnout limitations. We can't do it all, but it's likely we'll still try. I did. I don't wear a cape or sport a large 'S' on my chest. Bluntly speaking, cancer caregiving is hard and endless work. Some medical and psychology publications equate the anxiety of a cancer diagnosis for both the patient and spousal caregiver to PTSD (post-traumatic stress disorder).[25] [26] And that can even start before any of the real caregiving commences.

From my perspective, the expectation of caregiving was nothing more than fulfilling the promise I made about "in sickness and in health" on my wedding day. Caregiving needed to be done. The taking over of all housework while caregiving and working full time was a burden, no doubt. And I know I paid a steep price in my own health.

When you first learn that the person you love has cancer, eating and sleeping will likely be in short supply, which, among many other damaging results, will lessen your energy to carry out these new responsibilities. Prior to Shelley's December 2017 diagnosis, I was quite the stereotypical male in that I rarely cried over anything. But throughout those terrible initial weeks, my stomach ached with worry, and I lay awake in bed for hours on a nightly basis with the "tear faucets" seemingly set on full blast. I lost seven pounds that first week, and in the unhealthiest manner possible.

One evening in mid-January I felt so overwhelmed that I suddenly was overcome with shortness of breath, chest pains, dizziness, and rapid pulse. I thought I might be having a heart attack. Though Shelley had just undergone her third Adriamycin/Cytoxan chemo treatment the day before, she still managed to drive me to the hospital

ER, where I was later admitted for stress-induced atrial fibrillation. My erratic pulse was measured at 187 while my blood pressure was off the chart.

I was in the hospital overnight and had to stay well into the following day until my vital signs improved. The big conundrum was a vicious cause/effect cycle – I couldn't be discharged until I got my BP down and pulse rhythm back to normal. But on the other hand, the longer I was in the hospital and unable to be home taking care of Shelley, the more stress I experienced, which, of course, kept my BP up. Shelley had just finished chemo, and I perpetually worried that she needed me. Worse yet, as I heard and saw persistent, raucous coughing, it seemed that almost everyone in the ER, and subsequently on my floor when I was admitted, had the flu! Were I to have become infected, that could have been a disaster for Shelley. I wanted to get out of there much sooner than I was able, and, as I look back with some embarrassment, I was probably not the most cooperative patient for the poor medical staff to deal with.

That experience was without doubt a wakeup call. As I lay in my hospital bed, I kept saying to myself, "Keith, Shelley needs you now, more than ever. So you'd better unearth some coping mechanisms, and fast." As my friends had been constantly (and annoyingly) pestering me, they were absolutely right in that I would be no good to her if I couldn't take care of myself. While doing so was a gargantuan adjustment, I ultimately figured it out.

After I was discharged from the hospital, I found success in compartmentalizing life and caregiving duties more productively. Instead of only focusing on the big picture of cancer that included a potentially fatal outcome, I broke things down into dealing with smaller, more manageable pieces, one task at a time and one day at a time. When I was unable to keep up, I figured out how to ask others for help. This was actually easier than it sounds since most of our friends already contacted us regularly to offer their assistance. I began to take them up on their multiple offers. And I just gave myself an obligatory pass for not being perfect. When we had a good day, we counted it as a small victory. The more small victories we had in succession, the easier things were on the psychological side of coping. But even after I got out of the hospital, I still always politely declined when friends repeatedly offered to sit with Shelley so that I could take a day off. Shelley never got a day's reprieve, so why should I?

CHAPTER 7

The Culture of the Infusion Room

When I hear somebody sigh, "Life is hard," I am always tempt-ed to ask, "Compared to what?"

-Sydney Harris

After we first learned that cancer had invaded Shelley's body, it almost seemed incomprehensible that we would ever calm down from our initial fear and grief. But eventually it happened. As that new normal slowly became the *normal*, what was previously unexpected and un-known morphed into the predictable, routine, and, most important to us, our reaching a phase of acceptance. And that took place, in large part, because of the support we received from our oncology team.

It never occurred to me at the outset how strong the bonds of professional, but interpersonal, relationships we developed with *all* of our oncology team members would become. Throughout my life I've had good luck with the type of people my past and present physi-cians have been. Perhaps it's just the nature of the profession. I know that my brother is revered by his patients. But Shelley's and my expe-riences with our oncology people are just in a completely different stratosphere when it came to their empathy and understanding.

At times, they almost felt like family members.

I wrote earlier about my brief aggravation with the Christmas wishes given to patients as they left the clinic during our initial visit to Missouri Cancer Associates. But it was very short lived. Every employee treated us with kindness, respect, and empathy that terrible morning (and in every visit since). A few days after that first appointment, one of the MCA radiology nurses phoned us at home to confirm the time and date for Shelley's upcoming PET scan. Since Shelley was at work, I took the call. After I wrote down the requisite information, the nurse asked me how I was holding up. I suspect she'd heard a little concern and fear in my tone. "Not well," I half-whispered, while futilely attempting not to let my voice waver.

This nurse, who initially called only to briefly confirm an appointment, stayed on the line *for 15 minutes* consoling me. She revealed that she, too, was a breast cancer survivor, and not just once, but twice. She knew precisely what Shelley and I were going through. And she took the time to let us know that though she hadn't yet met us (she would, soon enough), she already knew the deep, dark intricacies of this ordeal. She empathized with our new reality, and, best of all, she offered hope. Talk about going the extra mile! She was beyond compassionate. As we looked past all the science and frustration over those uncontrolled recurrently dividing cells we call cancer, the experiential world of oncology seemed unparalleled in providing interpersonal support to those actually living the nightmare.

In fact, it wasn't just the oncologists, radiologists, and surgeons who seemed almost to befriend us. We even knew by first name the receptionists and appointment makers. But it was the nurses at Missouri Cancer Associates with whom we'd gotten closest. Those who drew Shelley's blood. Those who conducted preliminary consults before Dr. Makarian visited us in the exam room. The radiology nurses. And the infusion nurses.

God, *especially* the infusion nurses.

This is in no way to suggest that our chemo nurses were any better at their craft or in connecting with patients than the others. But because of the sheer frequency of treatment, our interactions with Nurse Lindsay and the others took place far more often and for longer periods of time.

Aside from our issues during Shelley's first chemotherapy of having to wait three hours for echocardiogram results and then the subsequent sickness later in the day, I can still honestly say that as we apprehensively walked into the infusion room for the first time, it was not *at all* what we expected it to be. We were both clearly struck by the positive culture. While some chemo recipients were sleeping or reading, others were involved, even energetically, in conversation with their caregivers and nurses, or with other patients and caregivers. The lighting in the room was pleasantly bright. There were televisions around the different infusion stations. The window sills were adorned with scores of those fun, silly gyrating solar-dancing toys that festively reflected various seasons and holidays. Much of everything looked, well, almost happy. In addition to the treatment bags, on many of the infusion poles faux containers were hanging that looked like whiskey, gin, and tequila bottles. In the venue of the most serious of medical treatments, the nurses were still able to add a little levity to which Shelley and I couldn't help but momentarily smile.

During Shelley's nearly five months of chemo treatment, we had our favorite nurse in Lindsay of course. But in reality she was likely no different than the others. They *all* cared about us, and given the fact that Shelley received chemo 16 times in that time period (which didn't include myriad other appointments in between), they got to know us pretty well. They often joked with us. In fun, they pleasantly argued with us about our professional sports team allegiances that reflected the fact that neither Shelley nor I grew up in Missouri. They complimented us when we were able to celebrate our small victories. They brought us coffee, food, treats, and various snacks that were available.

One day there were chocolate cupcakes. On another there was fresh fruit. Though the majority of our chemo sessions were in the early afternoon, there were some mornings when prepared fast-food breakfast sandwiches were sitting in the kitchen area for anyone to grab. I asked Lindsay if MCA provided everything. "We do the coffee, the protein drinks, and a few other things," she replied, "but a lot of people just randomly bring in treats and other food items on their own to share with the patients and caregivers."

I never asked specifically who those people were, but I knew that I one day wanted to become one of them. I wanted to give back once we reached the point that Shelley had beaten (a relative word in the world of oncology) her cancer.

I guess in some respects, the infusion room reflects positivity in the same way that parents often tell their small children after a knee scrape, "You're OK; there's no need to cry." Cancer, of course, is no minor scrape or bruise. But with nearly two million cases diagnosed in the U.S. each year, it's certainly not an uncommon occurrence either. And neither is treatment. Our nurses always projected the attitude that, while this was normal for them, our being there was their fight as much as ours, and that winning was the only option. They and our other oncology team members seemed to take it personally when there was a hiccup or backward step in this marathon. After Shelley's terrible reaction to the first treatment, the general attitude among everyone in the clinic was, *"We are going to fix this!"* And, lo and behold, there was very little nausea from that point forward that was related to chemotherapy.

We often referred to Nurse Lindsay as "our medical daughter." When she wasn't overly busy with other patients, she made a point of sitting down with us to talk during the slow, time-consuming infusion drips. She listened to us and laughed with us. She even cried with us on a couple of occasions when we were down. She was interested in seeing pictures of our family, in hearing how Karen's and Jake's wedding plans were evolving, and asking what we might be doing for an upcoming weekend. There was no question in my mind that she and the other infusion nurses tried to be this way with all their patients. Metaphorically, they were great in helping us get our minds off our scraped knees. Not only did interacting with them aid us psychologically, it helped pass the monotony of the 1-2 hours we were there. But mostly, they helped us maintain hope by making everything seem pretty standard, even when it wasn't. After a few weeks, the weekly or twice-weekly visits to MCA felt like a normal part of life.

In addition to regularly seeing the medical staff, many of the other patients became familiar faces to us as well. Some were further along in their treatment regimens. Others were just beginning. But everyone had a story. It seemed normal for people to talk and listen during treatment. Shelley was particularly good at connecting with other patients in the infusion room. She offered hope and empathy to those starting out who were still in the terrified-of-the-unknown stage. She also learned from others who were nearing the completion of their chemotherapy phase of treatment. The empathy seemed beneficial, if not crucial, to everyone as they coped through the sharing of their experiences. Yet, others were not so interested in talking, and I always respected their wishes. But sometimes all it took was a moment of mutual eye contact and reciprocal head nods that seemed to signify, "I hear you, brother, and I feel your pain."

Those receiving infusions always seemed supportive of one another in the infusion room, in the largest or even in the smallest of victories. On the December morning of Shelley's first treatment, a woman sitting in our section was completing her final chemotherapy infusion. At the finish, the nurses made a public announcement of this achievement, and both Shelley and I smiled and joined in the wild applause that took place. The nurses then provided her with a certificate of completion that they all had signed. Then they took instant-camera photos, and placed them on a special commemorative photo wall. When Shelley and I looked at the scores of completion photos, we didn't feel jealousy. We felt hope.

Obviously I can't say we looked forward to getting chemo each week. Even though the Taxol had a significantly less side-effect punch than the four Adriamycin/Cytoxan treatments, the cumulative effects over the course of months really wore on Shelley. But in our day-to-day new-normal reality, we coped, and we celebrated her small victories. And the multitude of interactions in the infusion room were very much a positive part of each of those weeks. Certainly it wasn't a happy place for everyone. But every effort was made for it to be as supportive as possible.

CHAPTER 8

The 12 Weeks of Taxol

Routine is important. I think a good routine diverts the mind from morbid imaginings.

-Grant Morrison

Thankfully, neither Shelley nor I became ill during the four and a half months of chemotherapy. Therefore, there was no, shall we say, "road construction" of infection to impede the chemo pathway while she progressed. Shelley's 12 Taxol treatments were stunningly simple in that they were repetitive and significantly more bearable than the four rounds of the Adriamycin/Cytoxan.

Of course, there's always more to the story. And I will be abundantly clear at the outset in saying that *nothing was easy about this treatment.* There were extended times when Shelley just felt terrible. But the nutshell version of these 12 weeks was that they were *almost* as predictable as normal life could be.

Each Friday from February 16 through May 4 possessed clockwork regularity. Because I had no scheduled classes that day of the week, I'd take Shelley to work in the morning, and she'd work a half day. I picked her up at noon, we went out to lunch near Missouri Cancer Associates, and then we drove over to the clinic for her 1:00 chemo appointment. After her blood was drawn and blood-count screenings were determined to be in the "normal" range, we usually got to the infusion room between 1:30 and 2:00. The Taxol treatment lasted about an hour. We'd return home circa 3:15 pm, and then she lay down for a one- to two-hour nap. Upon waking up, she'd feel refreshed, and we set out for our long-standing Friday-evening date night. This usually included dinner out and then often meeting up with friends at a local craft brewery for a beer and wonderful conversation. Most Friday evenings during Taxol treatments truly began our partial weekend escape from cancer.

On Saturdays, her energy level was still relatively high. We'd go shopping. Or for a hike, when she was able. Or to a local coffee house or winery. Whatever we did, we were definitely living for the now and enjoyed each moment we spent together when she felt able.

On Sunday mornings, however, the chemo-induced energy crash would arrive, and she'd be flat out on the couch for the majority of the day. By Monday morning she was still experiencing some fatigue, but she usually, with a few exceptions, felt well enough to return to work. And that was our weekly routine. For the most part, every weekend of the 12 was *predictable*. We could always hang our hats on that.

This is what you do when your spouse is fighting cancer. When the big-picture outcome is still in question. When there could be a metaphorical ticking timeclock hovering over us, measuring the finite number of remaining days during which she truly felt good. (Which, actually, is reality for us all, whether or not cancer is a part of our life equation.) When Shelley felt good *now*, we didn't waste the now by doing nothing. We set out to enjoy that time to its fullest.

If you're wondering how these feel-good events took place during a life-and-death battle with cancer, there are both short- and long-term answers. In part, Shelley was lucky not to have experienced any type of allergic reaction that is sometimes common with Taxol use. And that may have taken place, in part, because of a normal fire-prevention tactic from our oncology team. A portion of her weekly infusions contained quantities of an allergy medication. Since one of the typical side effects of that drug is drowsiness, there was a need for an immediate nap after her treatment. But an added steroid infusion provided what amounted to be about a 36-hour energy boost. Again, our oncology team's adjustments made chemo much more tolerable for Shelley.

Less potent chemotherapy is still chemotherapy. As the weeks progressed, slow-accumulating side-effects continued to build. Among them were hand and foot pain and neuropathy. This created issues for Shelley in finger dexterity (which was problematic in that her work required a lot of typing) and in walking. Walks and hikes, therefore, occurred less and less as Taxol treatment progressed. And while there are various medications to combat those conditions to an extent, the ensuing drugs often created after-effects of their own.

Gabapentin, for example, was used to help reduce pain and neuropathy in her hands and feet. But it often caused both constipation and diarrhea, for which laxatives and anti-diarrheal medications were needed. And each of those, obviously, counteracted the other. As a result, Shelley was taking multiple pills and capsules throughout the day, every day, which sometimes created stomach problems that required even more meds. It seemed to be an endless chain of side-effect drugs with each to treat the undesirable effects of the previous one.

Every week's conclusion kept the countdown-to-chemo-completion going at a steady pace. By March 9, Shelley reached the halfway mark as she finished her eighth round of the 16, and we began to see the light at the end of the tunnel. At that point, however, her fingernails and toenails were thickening, softening, loosening, and turning, as she would say, an ugly dark brown color. She would eventually lose a couple of those nails. But a little polish here and there seemed to keep them temporarily out of sight and therefore out of mind. The Sunday energy crashes became more pronounced, making the Monday recuperation more and more strenuous. As we expected, chemotherapy's snowballing effects were clearly taking their toll.

Predictability, while helpful in our knowing what to expect, certainly didn't alleviate any of the physical issues and symptoms that continued to worsen with the passage of each treatment.

March 30 was particularly notable in that, prior to Shelley receiving her 11th treatment, Dr. Makarian *could not manually find the tumor!* We were ecstatic! Of course, we knew there would be some sort of radiological view to determine its exact size and position prior to any post-chemo surgery. And we remembered my brother's sage medical advice of not letting ourselves get too emotionally up or down during the journey. But the fact that the tumor couldn't be detected by hand seemed to be an awfully good indicator that the chemotherapy was indeed doing its job.

Treatment number 13 coincidentally took place on Friday the 13th in April. This was a particularly fun evening for Shelley in that good friends Lorena and Cinnamon took her out for a fun ladies night. They went to get a pedicure where they got foot massages, a sugar-scrub on their legs and feet, a toenail trim, and beautiful polish on their toenails. Of course, Shelley got her favorite color, teal. Then the three of them went out for dinner before meeting up for a drink with their husbands. It was a wonderful get-together for all six of us. At this point, Shelley only had three chemotherapy treatments remaining, with the final one targeted for May 4.

The day before her penultimate infusion, Shelley attended an appointment with her surgeon, Dr. Peterson, on April 26 to discuss tumor removal options. Since the chemo was clearly working to reduce tumor size, Shelley, in consultation with the surgeon, decided on a lumpectomy. Wishing to avoid potential reconstruction complications from a mastectomy, a lumpectomy was exactly what Shelley was hoping for. Surgery was scheduled for Friday, June 1.

Radiation would likely follow sometime in July and August, which we hoped would conclude all treatment. Of course at this point we didn't know how this was going to play itself out. But with only one chemo and a less invasive operation to go, we were feeling *much* better about everything than we were just four months prior.

May the fourth be with you!

Unofficially known as *Star Wars* day for its obvious play on words with a line from the classic 1977 film, May 4, 2018 was an important milestone in Shelley's and my respective family trees: It was her parents' 55th wedding anniversary, and it also marked what would have been my late mother's 95th birthday.

But we will long remember it for being the day of Shelley's concluding chemo infusion and the wonderful celebration that followed. Since and including that terrible December 21 treatment, she had endured this chemical madness 16 times. She had lost her hair, but not her beauty. She had lost dexterity in her hands and fingers, but not her ability to lovingly caress her husband. She lost some energy, but not her positive attitude and bubbly demeanor. She said she had temporarily lost a little mental function from chemo brain, but not her ability to love and feel emotion.

In describing situations that test human limits, my eloquent niece so simply, but profoundly, liked to say, "Invictus, baby!" [Invictus is Latin for "unconquerable" or "undefeated."] We adopted it as our signature line as well. Finishing chemotherapy would be such a colossal milestone. Therefore, it was time for a celebration of exceptional magnitude. So there had to be some conniving and manipulative efforts on the part of Shelley's husband to organize a special surprise. I conspired with some of my best friends in the world – who also work with me at Westminster College – to gather at Missouri Cancer Associates for a surprise group congratulations. We were so pleased that Karen and Jake took the afternoon off from their respective jobs and traveled all the way from Kansas City to partake in the surprise and festivities.

Many participants brought with them an array of clever congratulatory and motivational signs, posters, and balloons. In addition, they all wore special pink buttons I previously ordered that said, *#ShelleyStrong*. And I had a pink T-shirt made for Shelley with a caricature of a woman sporting a "Fight like a girl" tattoo, and included the text, "I finished 16 rounds of chemotherapy. And I took it like a woman. #ShelleyStrong."

At 3:00 pm, Shelley's final infusion-ending bell rang out. And right after the needle was removed from her port, I led the surprise contingent into the chemotherapy room, and we began chanting, "Shelley strong! Shelley strong!" Of course, she was completely blown away in surprise. There were many happy tears, and even a few from her husband. She put on her new shirt and received her Missouri Cancer Associates chemo-completion certificate. Shelley, Karen, Jake, and I posed for some photos that included a few members of the wonderful MCA nursing staff.

After the surprise at MCA, we all moved the celebration to imbibe at our favorite downtown Columbia hangout, where we were happily joined by Nick (who, unfortunately, had class until 4:00, and couldn't be with us for the surprise). We drank good beer and wine, made heartfelt toasts, and simply reveled in the timeless, celebratory moments. Chemo. Was. *Done!*

Next would be surgery, radiation, and hormonal therapy, so the long road would still continue. But on that May 4th day, our cry was *Invictus, baby!* As we all knew, Shelley truly demonstrated herself to be an unconquerable, courageous, and resilient soul.

CHAPTER 9

Surgery Means No More Secrets

Moment of truth. Are you ready?

-Randy Jackson

Though I've had several "procedures," I've never, as of this writing, experienced anything that was medically classified as surgery. The idea of someone taking a sharp scalpel, cutting through flesh and muscle tissue, and then removing a part of the anatomy that was naturally and purposely placed by human biology admittedly makes me a little squeamish. With anesthesia and other drugs playing a major role, there seems to be much that could go wrong. Thankfully, my intellectual side recognizes the positive return over the low risk factor of routine operations. It would be sheer repetition for an outstanding and well qualified surgeon like Dr. Peterson to get in and get out with the least amount of invasiveness. And in the case of cancer surgery, all risks aside, there is an open door to actually see what cancer is doing and to assess the effectiveness of treatment on the malignancy. Not to mention that we wanted that damn tumor out of her body once and for all!

Surgery for Shelley would ultimately provide long-awaited answers to our many questions regarding her progress. All manual indicators were that pretty much everything had gone precisely the way

Dr. Makarian had hoped. But the June 1 operation was going to allow for a quick and impending moment of truth. Shelley would have what remained of her tumor and the closest lymph node adjacent to the tumor (often called a sentinel lymph node) removed. Visually, the surgeon could see the overall extent of how well – or poorly – the chemo affected the tumor. Even more importantly, we needed to know if there was progression on the microscopic level.

Since unchecked cancer cells from a primary breast tumor normally travel first to a nearby sentinel node, removing it could eventually tell us if the malignancy had been stopped in its tracks by way of pathology testing. The process involves cutting the extracted node into microscopic slices and viewing each one for any residual cancer cells. If there were none, there was a good chance the chemo killed all of the cancer. Radiation would still proceed to target any potentially remaining cells within her breast tissue, but this would be the *best* possible outcome. It would take several days of testing after surgery for the pathology report to materialize.

June 1 turned out to be a long and trying day. Frazzled nerves were the likely culprit when I woke up at 2:45 am. After about 10-15 minutes of anxious and fully-conscious restlessness, I realized there was little chance of getting back to sleep. So I decided to head out for an early start on my daily morning walk.

The nighttime darkness was calming as I proceeded. There were very few cars out and about, and the serene peace and quiet allowed me opportunity to try to clear my head of some pessimistic fears I'd begun to harbor since the euphoria of the May 4 chemo finale. But worrying, something I happen to be very good at, wasn't going to change the day's outcome, one way or the other. Author Karen Salmansohn once wrote, "Worrying doesn't stop the bad stuff from happening. It just stops you from enjoying the good stuff."[27] And there was strong reason to believe good stuff would be taking place this day, that the surgery would reveal our nightmare to soon be over. I wouldn't allow myself to get overconfident, but there was no question I felt that the prospect for a good outcome seemed legitimate, if not inevitable.

The beginning of June is ever so close to summer solstice, so it wasn't surprising to see a hint of pre-sunrise twilight glow seeping over the eastern horizon when I returned home at about 4:30 am. Shelley was still fast asleep, and I decided to make some coffee and quietly have breakfast before she got up. She'd been directed not to eat anything after midnight prior to her morning surgery, so I didn't want her to see me eating since she likely would be hungry when she awoke at 5:30.

We showered, got dressed, and drove to the hospital. We arrived at the specified check-in time of 7:00 am so that Shelley could have an ultrasound and a wire marking line installed for the surgeon to see precisely where the tumor was. A mammogram and a nuclear medicine CT scan were also conducted as part of the process.

With Dr. Peterson at the helm, Shelley's surgery began at about 11:00. Nick arrived in the waiting area not long after. A couple of other friends graciously joined us for added support. Though it seemed like a much longer wait, the operation was finished in 90 minutes, which was precisely the general timeframe initially given to us. We were told it would still take Shelley an hour or two to recover from the anesthesia.

At about 1:15 pm, Dr. Peterson emerged and called me over to provide an update. I was heartened to see that she was *smiling*! Nick and I sat with her for a few minutes in the consult room. Her exact opening words were, "Based on the visuals, it definitely appears the chemotherapy did its job." Both Nick and I loudly exhaled. She told us she removed what was left of the tumor along with an adjacent lymph node. "The visuals of the node also look encouraging," she said. "But of course, we're sending it to pathology for a microscopic view to be certain, and we should get the results sometime next week. In the meantime, it'll be another hour before you can see her, but she's doing just fine."

As a well-educated college professor of speech and rhetoric, I'd like to think I'm at least somewhat articulate in vividly describing situations deserving of aesthetic eloquence. But the only words I could find to outwardly express my exhilaration at the moment were, "Oh, wow!" I probably repeated them, to no one in particular, several times over.

Nick and I returned to the waiting room and gleefully began texting the updated news to family members and friends. Karen had gotten off work early and arrived from Kansas City soon after, and suffice to say, we were all feeling quite good about everything at the moment. We couldn't wait to see Shelley.

We sat in the waiting room for another hour and a half when a nurse approached us to say that Shelley was having a bad reaction to the anesthesia, and that she had been throwing up repeatedly. We were able to go in to see her at that point, but she was clearly not feeling well. It was a grim reminder of that first chemo treatment back in December. We needed to wait several hours longer before she felt well enough to go home. Though the surgery was finished at 12:30, we weren't able to leave the hospital until 7:45 pm. Sadly, she vomited three more times upon our return home before she fell asleep for the night. As I previously said, it was a *very* long day.

While the preliminary outlook appeared encouraging, I had to keep reminding myself that cancer is a sneaky assassin. Conceivably, there could be a need for more surgery, the pathology report could have bad results, and there were other unknown factors that could paint a negative picture. We knew it was best to be patient and not to let our emotions get too high or too low. But, unquestionably, we had just cleared another major hurdle.

The next few days were spent at home in recovery from the anesthesia and normal post-operative pain. Shelley spent a lot of time lying down, but she noticeably improved each day. By June 5, she expressed a strong desire to get out of the house "to go *anywhere*," so we decided to kill two birds with one stone and do a little needed grocery shopping. We quickly wrote up a food list and drove to the grocery store a couple of miles from our home.

We were waiting at a stoplight before pulling into the store parking lot when Shelley's phone rang. It was Dr. Peterson's office on caller ID. Of course, we were anticipating this call to learn of the pathology results – promising results, we'd hoped.

Shelley hesitated for a moment as we both knew how this routine often went down: If it were good news, the call would come from a nurse, an assistant, or a receptionist. But with bad news, it would likely be our surgeon on the line to convey it. After about five rings, Shelley finally answered.

"Hi, Shelley, it's Dr. Peterson. Do you have time to talk?"

CHAPTER 10

I Exhaled When
I Shouldn't Have

Cancer reminds me of a very bad but tenacious performer who, although no one wants to see, insists on doing an encore, having a return engagement, making a comeback and, worst of all, going on tour.

-Valerie Harper

After Shelley's June 1 surgery, we knew the tumor was gone. With the removed lymph node initially appearing to be cancer free, all we needed was a clean pathology report on that sentinel node. For three days, we reveled in the seeming likelihood that we were in the home stretch; that radiation would be the final lap of this dreadful cancer journey; that by early to mid-autumn, we'd be where we were prior to the start of this terrible nightmare.

"It's truly about over," I remember thinking. I exhaled in relief.

It turned out to be a brash, premature thought on my part.

Dr. Peterson's June 5 phone call alerted us with information we hoped we wouldn't hear. The pathology report revealed isolated cancer cells remaining in the lymph node, which necessitated more extensive surgery just three days later on June 8 for an axillary dissection to remove more nodes. The tumor was gone, of course, and that was something to be pleased with. But, again, cancer builds on the microscopic level. Even one remaining cell could eventually produce a new life-threatening tumor. "Cancer-free" only means no detectable malignant cells. Regrettably, Shelley still had some cancer lingering in her beaten-up body.

Probably eight more lymph nodes were removed from under Shelley's arm in the June 8 surgery. On the plus side, a change made to her anesthesia had far better results. She was able to go home soon after initial recovery without any vomiting. On the minus side, this was a more complex operation with greater pain and extended recovery.

With fewer remaining nodes to filter and clear away lymphatic fluid, the surgery included the temporary implant of a so-called Jackson-Pratt tube under the arm for drainage into an exterior rubber syringe. We had to empty it a couple of times a day. In addition, the inserted connecting tube regularly poked into Shelley's area muscle tissue causing her numerous unexpected sharp, painful jabs until it was removed about two weeks later. This constantly interrupted her sleep during that time as well.

We still had the possibility of a good outcome if all the removed nodes were cancer-free. With so many to check, it took pathology almost two weeks to get the results to us. But on June 20, it was again Dr. Peterson who phoned Shelley to tell her that seven of the eight nodes contained individual cancer cells. Detectable cancer was still in her body.

What we learned in a follow-up consultation with our oncologist was that even with some remaining cancer cells in the lymph nodes, there was still a possibility for a complete remission with subsequent treatment. But it also indicated a higher risk of cancer recurrence. There was a reasonable chance that everything could be fine, but not as likely as if the nodes had come back clean.

I've long used the term "microscopic terrorist" as an analogy to describe individual cancer cells. I guess it seems appropriate in that the Department of Homeland Security uses the word "cell" to describe very small, hidden terrorist groups. Cancer doesn't need to "recruit" other terrorist cells, however. It simply manufactures them through rapid and uncontrolled cell division that is often asymptomatic. Until it's too late. And much like Kyle Reese described Arnold Schwarzenegger's cyborg character in the movie *The Terminator*, cancer "can't be bargained with, it can't be reasoned with, it doesn't feel pity or remorse or fear."[28] It can just keep coming.

Though no one ever witnesses the initial development phase of cancer, malignant tumors probably begin as a single mutated strand of DNA within one cell out of the trillions of cells that make up our individual bodies. Technology just isn't there to detect that one cell.

After speaking with our oncologist, the plan was to continue with hormonal therapy (tamoxifen) and to follow through with the scheduled six weeks of radiation when Shelley completely recovered from surgery. The one change that would take place was that she would also be put on an oral chemotherapy regimen for six months. This meant new chemicals and new side effects (and their accumulations), though they wouldn't be nearly as pronounced as her traditional chemo treatments. Again, no chemo is easy. The reasonable hope was that this combination would, perhaps in almost napalm-bomb-like fashion, kill all of the remaining cancer cells she still had.

Throughout treatment, our good friends had constantly posted, texted, and emailed positive, cliché messages for Shelley and me to keep smiling, to hang in there, to keep our chins up, to stay strong, and to be positive. But we just weren't interested in reading them on that day. So I uploaded a note on CaringBridge suggesting that this was not the best time to offer any cheerleading philosophies. Or to advise us on how to feel or what to think. Or to ask numerous questions about this painful revelation. It was time for them to step back and let us temporarily grieve. And, if they wanted, to just listen. To hear us. To co-grieve. And that's precisely what they did.

Temporary grieving was not only a necessary part of our coping process, it was vital in order for us to come to terms with and, ultimately, get past the defeats we would have. Our anguish didn't mean we'd given up, that we'd thrown in the towel, or that we'd conceded anything.

It did, however, mean that we're human. Gone was the hope that we were in the home stretch of treatment. This game wasn't just going into overtime or extra innings. It became a new game. As one of our CaringBridge followers appropriately wrote, there are times that crappy things happen in our lives that we simply can't control, and our natural emotions of fear, sadness, and disappointment not only kick in, they briefly take over. Sometimes we need a day or three just to be exhausted. And sad. And furious at the unfairness when life doesn't simply throw us a curveball but instead changes the game entirely. But those moments are important in that they let us take a breath, regroup, and return to the battle again the next day. Or the day after that. Shelley and I had to rediscover the physical and emotional resolve to continue her terrible fight. We needed time to adjust our collective mindset to this new, unexpected change in our reality. And that would soon happen. But not on that day.

Through their supporting words, delivering prepared meals, and often helping with our job duties among other things, our friends and family had been a steadying force for us. Time after time, they extended hands to help us up during the numerous occasions we'd been knocked down. They did so much to help absorb our pain. Shelley and I understood that though this was our unfortunate experience to cope with, they were still the biased spectators sitting on the edges of their stadium or arena seats. They were watching and rooting for us, gritting their teeth over each referee call, agonizing over every boxing round, inning, and quarter. We knew they anticipated medical news almost as much as we did.

After all the boxing analogies we'd used over the months to describe the blows we thought we'd dealt Shelley's tumor, it turned out that cancer delivered a haymaking sucker punch of its own. And it was one that left us both emotionally reeling.

CHAPTER 11

When Well-Meaning People Say It All Wrong

I've learned that people will forget what you said, people will forget what you did, but people will never forget how you made them feel.

-Maya Angelou

Oh my goodness. As I look back at some of the inane things I've said to cancer fighters over my lifetime, I sometimes wonder how I still have them and their families as friends. I always felt the necessity to use my words for putting an upbeat spin on their life-or-death situations. I remember saying things I once thought were beneficial for friends who were going through cancer themselves or with a loved one. I conveyed sympathy and hope. I extended my thoughts and best wishes. I made general, hollow-sounding "Let me know if you need anything" offers of help. I would chime in, using the most positive of vocal tones: "Be strong." As if they had some sort of choice when their lives were on the line. "Don't worry. You're going to be fine." "Keep fighting. You'll get through this." All of these must have sounded as if I were making their very realistic fears seem unjustified. What I couldn't fathom at the time was the sheer terror they were experiencing from the endless medical fallout of a life-threatening diagnosis.

I thought it's what they *wanted* to hear. But only after my wife was diagnosed years later, and a handful of friends and colleagues started saying the same things I previously said (and with the same positive intentions), did I realize how mindless – even manifestly stupid – many of those words must have sounded to the cancer families I tried to comfort in the past.

In the immortal words of *Seinfeld* character George Constanza, yadda … yadda … yadda.

There is no question that the aims of all our family, friends, colleagues, and acquaintances were laser focused on their trying to help us. I *know* that. They care deeply for us, and when they learned of our new heartbreaking circumstances, they, too, were emotionally impacted and involved. The vast majority of them seemed to know precisely what to say. But a few others said things completely wrong.

The term *general semantics* refers to the study of words, meaning, and their interpretations by listeners. And those interpretations can evoke emotion. Since I teach college-level communication courses, I am, by trade, a semanticist. The words we choose to describe our thoughts will have much to do with how we (and our messages) are perceived. Empathic listening is quite helpful when listeners have similar life events to reflect on and are therefore able to "walk a mile in another's shoes." But short of their having gone through the experience of being a caregiver or treated for cancer, they truly have no full understanding of what it's like. Empathy can be tough in that circumstance. They can vicariously imagine of course. However, they can't accurately sense or assess the totality of what we're feeling. That can sometimes make it difficult for them to articulate things that don't come off as unintentionally insensitive. And this can sometimes happen when acquaintances give advice they are probably not qualified to give.

There was certainly one bit of guidance many gave that sounded silly to me at the outset, but which turned out to be absolutely right:

"Keith, you're no good as a caregiver if you don't take care of yourself!" The problem was that their message felt more like nagging than anything else. I always did the best I could. But my experience in caregiving for the one I love was often an emotional deluge. My internal stress level made eating and sleeping extremely difficult, which, of course, would eventually render very unhealthy outcomes if not kept in check. But pestering me to take care of myself was a little like telling a chain-smoker (who desperately wants to quit but doesn't know how) that "You need to stop smoking." Taking care of oneself is much easier said than done when you're not the one saddled with the physical and emotional strain of caregiving, of wondering about your spouse's long-term health, of having to keep up with employment responsibilities though you sometimes need to care for your partner 24/7. Not so easy to do when you actually have those burdens.

A normal reaction for close, desperate friends is to want to do or say anything they can to help the cancer family. But what is helpful, and what is not? Unfortunately, the answer can be rather complicated. The friends may find themselves in a dilemma of determining the proper balance between inserting their communication efforts to aid, while not intruding on the family's periodic need for privacy. For the cancer family, keeping friends at arm's length may cause them to assume their help is not wanted. And this could happen at the time we might need them most. So, in our prison of overwhelming emotion, we had to be particularly aware of how we responded to their good intentions. Nick has told me on several occasions, "Dad, they're just trying to be nice. It might be best to keep your mouth filter on." Sage advice, indeed.

Knowing the right things to say to us was sometimes (and understandably) quite elusive to some who'd never experienced cancer in their own families. Just as I had done in the past, some mistakenly shared positive words and perceptions in the belief that it would make the cancer and our fight against it less frightening, less distressing, and more tolerable.

I quickly learned it doesn't work that way.

I've also heard and read many cancer survivors and caregivers who've stated that the only thing worse than their friends and co-workers saying things in insensitive ways would be for them to say nothing at all. It's much like teachers who tell their students that there are no dumb questions.

As a cancer caregiver and a career college teacher, I just might occasionally disagree on both counts. I find that students receiving a new assignment without reading it often ask me, for example, about due dates, paper length, source requirements, theme, and other in-formation already made painfully clear in the assignment sheet and even on the syllabus. Those aren't good questions; they're lazy ques-tions, and they do waste class time. And if someone says nothing to a cancer family, it doesn't mean they don't care about us. I appreciated colleagues' well wishes when they materialized, but I wasn't keeping tabs on who did or did not extend them.

Certainly no one at work *owed* me any condolences. But I'll also admit that I was initially surprised (though not negatively) by the reticence of three colleagues, professors I'd worked with for many years. I wouldn't consider them to be close, off-campus friends. They are professional associates, good people with whom I've served on a committee or two, but who have said nothing to me about Shelley since her diagnosis. It couldn't be that they didn't know. I've been very public in disseminating information to all who have asked for updates. I even decorated my office door in pink with adorning breast cancer ribbons and photos of Shelley. But those colleagues, whose offices are on my floor, have not said anything beyond an occasional "Good morning, Keith" or short work-related discussion when literally everyone else has. Perhaps they truly wanted to say something but just couldn't find the right words. And that was definitely OK by me. One of my good friends who is currently fighting an aggressive form of breast cancer put it this way:

> "How people approach you [as a cancer-fighter or caregiver] is most likely a reflection of their ability (or inability) to cope, not a reflection of how much they care. This is a tough lesson, and you have every right to feel hurt and angry if a loved one distances themselves from you during a time when you need them to step forward. People make themselves scarce for a lot of reasons, many of which say nothing about their feelings for you. Some people are in denial; they can't handle the thought of possibly losing you, so they pretend nothing is happening. Others desperately want to reach out but are terrified of saying or doing the wrong thing, so they say and do nothing. Still others become scared and sad because the diagnosis brings out their own fears of mortality, leading them to avoid the topic — or you — entirely."[29]

On the positive side, it made for three fewer people taking time to have me revisit and rehash painful information. It meant three fewer people who might have shared well-meaning thoughts that could have been worded in unhelpful approaches. At worst, it's an even tradeoff. And I don't hold it against them in the least. Like me, they each had the drama of their own worlds to deal with.

There is much disagreement regarding the dos and don'ts – or, as my colleague and cancer survivor, Mari, calls them, the dos and taboos – of communicating with cancer patients and their family caregivers. But I have two all-purpose, can't miss, don't-violate-these-*ever* recommended axioms to share: First, no one should, overtly or covertly, treat our cancer situation as if they're part-owner. And second, no one should *ever* tell survivors or caregivers how to feel or react to their plight.

My family's cancer story isn't about anyone but us. It doesn't concern anyone's religious or philosophical convictions but ours. It's no one else's tragedy to frame or to cope with or to make decisions about. We would *love* to relinquish ownership. But, quite unfortunately, cancer unceremoniously and indelibly rammed itself into our lives.

I teach my students that communication receivers – listeners and readers of information directed to them – have an inherent duty to try to interpret messages the way they were truly intended. Simultaneously, senders – speakers and writers – have an equal responsibility to word their messages as accurately, effectively, and appropriately as possible. However, when the emotional stress of cancer is thrown into the mix, those pragmatic rules can be very difficult to follow. Shelley and I quickly found our own objectivity and a sense of perspective to be the first casualties of a new cancer diagnosis.

Coping with the torrent of well-wishers was, at times, daunting. Nevertheless, it still was comforting to know that Shelley and I had so many people who gave a damn about us. But try as they might, there were some who just weren't very good with their words, and *we had to accept that*. As a result, I eventually found that our family fared best if we could simply "hear" the message those friends truly intended to say: "We care about you; we hurt for you; we want to be there to help you if there's anything you need from us," even when the words they used were clumsy or ill-expressed. Most of the time – not always, but most of the time – we've been successful at doing that.

The following are some of the more lamentable – though needless to say, well meaning – and sometimes even eye-rolling comments we received during our cancer journey, along with my internal reactions that, for the most part, I managed to quell (again, thank you, Nick) with my mouth filter. I will elaborate on a few of them in the coming pages.

1) *"I believe everything happens for a reason."* Of course, some things really *do* happen for specific reasons. Some auto accidents take place because a driver has been drinking, or speeding, or texting, or falling asleep at the wheel. Employees are often fired explicitly because they do substandard work. But the "everything happens for a reason" line for cancer patients seems to do little but reach for some sort of artificial, pre-destination justification. And I don't think it's *ever* helpful to philosophically rationalize human suffering.

2) *"God has a plan for you, and He doesn't give you any burden He knows you can't handle."* I'm not trying to disrespect anyone's religious convictions. Admittedly, I don't really have a firm possession of religious faith. Though I'd consider myself to be more of a hopeful agnostic than anything, I *can* say I'm definitely not an atheist. Therefore, I think it's highly doubtful that God woke up one morning and randomly thought, "Gee, I think Shelley and Keith Hardeman need a life lesson on marital strength and character development, so I'm gonna give her cancer and watch them hopefully figure it out." Neither Shelley nor I believe for a nanosecond that God intentionally inflicts anyone with cancer. I'm pretty sure He has far more pressing things on His plate to deal with, such as war, murder, famine, and large-scale social and economic injustice.

3) *"You need a better attitude."* Hey, we did our best throughout treatment, but sometimes it just isn't possible to perpetually simulate things going well when they're not. And, as I will discuss in a bit, there's really no proven correlation between attitude and cancer survival rate.

4) *"Is that the good kind or the bad kind of cancer to have?"* While some forms of cancer are less aggressive and dangerous than others, I can assure you that there's truly no "good kind" of cancer. I cannot accurately express the depth of how

much I wish this question would never be asked of anyone with a malignancy.

5) *"Chemotherapy is poison, so you should be using alternative therapies, instead."* Well, that's probably half correct. Chemo *is* poison. But alternative "therapies" really don't offer any empirical curative evidence. It's anecdotal at best. Conventional treatments such as chemo, radiation, and surgery don't always work, either. But, comparatively, there's much more clear and scientific evidence that they often do.

6) *"Keith, I am convinced that optimistic thoughts will positively affect the results of her upcoming mammogram."* I know this comment was meant to allay my anticipatory concern about the results of an important approaching test. Call me a pessimist, but I'm far more pragmatic than that. I am patently annoyed by the trendy sports saying, "It is what it is." But it may be the best descriptor in capturing the essence of austere cancer realities. When we have an MRI, a PET scan, a mammogram, or a biopsy, it provides a small window to see what already is or isn't inside of Shelley's body. Cancer is either there or it isn't, independent of what our preferred test outcome may be. If it does exist, optimistic thoughts amount only to wishing the malignancy to simply go away prior to a test. And if it's already there, those thoughts can't change the fact.

7) *"Maybe you should change physicians/clinics."* Shelley was being treated at a distinguished cancer center, so I honestly didn't know how to respond to this. While shaking my head, I silently let it go into one ear and right out the other as Shelley spent precious energy on the phone trying to respectfully defend and explain to her good and well-meaning friend the patently obvious.

8) *"My friend's mother died from that kind of cancer."* OK, perhaps that was his way of showing us he understood the gravity

of Shelley's diagnosis. But we were already in full-throttle-awareness mode of cancer's prospective fatal outlook. We didn't really need to be reminded. Again.

9) *"You should be happy it's not stage IV."* Shelley's breast cancer was typed at stage IIIA, meaning it had spread well into her lymphatic system. True, it wasn't stage IV, but stage III cancer is certainly nothing to be comparatively celebrated. This idealist utterance clearly violated the "Please don't tell us how to react to our cancer" axiom.

10) *"Oh Keith, relax. She's gonna be fine."* Idealism, again, at its worst. Obviously, this was meant to inspire hope, confidence, and reduce anxiety. But it seemed to be more of a tone-deaf response than anything. When I'm asked to explain what is happening to my wife's body, and the individual then proceeds to tell me not to worry and that all will be just fine, it only dismisses my legitimate fears.

I've read many articles containing thoughtful advice on how to respond to a family dealing with the crisis of a cancer diagnosis or other life-threatening condition. While I don't always agree with all suggestions, they do give me pause and opportunity to reflect on how I might help others and how I react to those trying to help us. The more options I have from which to choose in my communication repertoire, the better chance I have of selecting the most appropriate ones for specific individuals. Predictably, when I get down to the comment sections of said articles, I often see a wide range of spirited disagreement, and, sadly, some remarks are even worded in far less than gracious terms. But that's only indicative of the fact that what works for one cancer family may not work for another. It's proof positive that there is no magic-bullet comment, no single correct thing to say or do across the board that would please everyone.

To those who truly want to help folks like Shelley and me, I suggest trying to assess, in advance, how a cancer family might react to various statements. In other words, as all communication professors say to their students, it is important to know one's audience and to analyze their needs before speaking to them about something as sensitive as their cancer. We're all different, and there's often a very fine line between saying something supportive and expressing words that could be perceived as hurtful or even offensive.

When friends and co-workers try to turn crappy into happy

Why?

Why?

Why do some people seem to have this irrepressible compulsion to outwardly insist that we always look at the bright side of everything, no matter how grave or critical the situation is? There are multiple approaches toward benevolently expressing thoughts of concern, but those mindless crappy-to-happy sentiments kept coming our way throughout the journey. And well-meaning as they were intended, they were truly some of the most awkward and insensitive things people said to us.

As previously stated, upon learning about Shelley's diagnosis, our professional and personal contacts clearly felt a great deal of our emotional pain. We appreciated their strong desire to remove some of the sting from what was happening. I guess the thought was that if their words helped us think about the situation differently, it would somehow make things better. But that isn't possible. *Words can't take cancer away.*

Contrived, philosophical, or spiritual spin almost seems to glorify someone else's agonizing, dire circumstance. These philosophical witticisms often miscalculate the magnitude of our life-and-death struggle, and hearing them applied to our story never made us feel better about having cancer. One woman, whose mother was fighting breast cancer, described others' unsolicited attempts at perceptual influencing this way: "I feel it is very important that each person is able to follow their own path in how they deal with breast cancer and what feels right for them. Any ... friend or family member needs to listen to their wishes and not pressure them down another road."[30]

I very much agree. I think it's best to just allow cancer fighters and caregivers to be the ones who, if need be, exclusively create their own philosophies and for their friends to strictly abide by them. Even those directly affected by cancer don't always agree with one another, which is perfectly fine. For instance, I've heard a number of patients powerfully describe their ideas that cancer has almost eruditely taught them about love, appreciation, and life perception. They've stressed that the disease can help us all to learn how to enjoy the moment and not to sweat the little things that pale by comparison. I certainly appreciate and respect that as a valid point of view when they apply it to their own cancer stories. Whatever works for them, works. For them.

I, on the other hand, just never had that kind of philosophical epiphany. Perhaps it would be better if I had. But to me, cancer is wholly unworthy of even the slightest of gratitude or praise. I see it as one thing, and one thing only: a vicious, cold-blooded killer. And that is all. I'll never perceive it as any type of teacher or character builder. I staunchly refuse to give Shelley's cancer the least bit of credit for spawning anything beyond total life upheaval any more than I would give life-lesson recognition to a kidnapper or terrorist holding a loaded gun to her head. Conclusions I may have come to about revamping personal priorities after her diagnosis were of my individual creation, not cancer's. Then, again, this is but my own perspective. And I am known in my crowd for being a bit of a pessimist at times.

Occasionally and sadly, I have felt the need to remove the mouth filter, to be blunt in telling a few people that not only was what they said unhelpful, it had crossed the line into being inappropriate. As an example, when the end of treatment was only a few weeks away, someone suggested to me that "When Shelley beats this, the two of you might actually look back someday and see the cancer experience as a gift to your marriage."

Insert eye roll.

"Not an ice cream cone's chance in Hades would I ever think anything remotely close," I bluntly responded with an adamant tone and a wry smile. Yes, as I just disclosed, I can be a pessimist. But hear me out on this one.

Few, if any, of us would be so insensitive as to tell rape victims that their attack was some sort of gift, that all they need is a good attitude, that everything happens for a reason, and that they should see the violence, brutality, emotional distress, and physical injuries of their sexual assault as a constructive learning experience. So why would we subject cancer fighters to that sort of "logic"? In my care-giving observations, I can state with the utmost of certainty that we found *absolutely nothing* redeeming about anything my wife has gone through and the myriad ways her body has been breached and assaulted throughout her treatment. I told the individual that during the course of over a year, Shelley was faced with:

- having highly toxic chemicals injected into her chest for an hour or more nearly every week for the better part of five months;
- needles frequently piercing her arms, hands, and chest;
- violent episodes of vomiting;
- losing all of her head and body hair, including eyebrows and eyelashes;
- her fingernails and toenails weakening while turning brown and black;
- losing some of those nails in the process;
- enduring severe pain and constant neuropathy in her hands and feet;

- having her body repeatedly cut open with parts of it taken out and things put into it;
- experiencing long-lasting post-surgical pain;
- emptying lymph fluid from her Jackson-Pratt drain through her surgical incision on a daily basis for two weeks along with the constant pain of the drain tube moving about and poking inside her muscle tissue;
- suffering endless fatigue;
- braving the gut-wrenching urgency of waiting on pins and needles for doctors' phone calls that would reveal highly anticipated, but equally feared and potentially dreaded, test results;
- spending hours almost every week waiting in hospitals and clinics;
- undergoing painful physical therapy after surgery for weeks on end to regain strength, flexibility, and mobility to perform the simplest of movements and tasks;
- withstanding concentrated radiation entering her body on a daily basis for six weeks, painfully irritating her skin and breast tissue;
- sharing ownership of her body with physicians, nurses, students, and other medical strangers who constantly scrutinize, touch, poke, and prod her naked breast.
- having to watch her husband observing the endless physical and emotional suffering of the person he loves most in the world and being powerless to help her.

For many cancer fighters, this, and far worse, is their normal. How would any of this, I asked, sound like some sort of desired keepsake?

During a TV talk show, a noted interviewer asked a celebrity if his incurable disease (not cancer) could be seen as a gift.[31] The celebrity politely responded that, if so, it's "a gift that keeps on taking." I used that very line in response to my acquaintance. I continued by telling him that even if one day my wife were ultimately cured, our lives, undeniably, would have been far better without the experience than with it. We're not better or stronger or more loving people because of it.

While many will disagree, cancer, to us, is not about character development. It's a slog – a protracted fight for survival while slowly crawling through physical and emotional hell. Throughout Shelley's 14 months of treatment, I wore a button every day that read, "Cancer sucks," because plainly and simply, *cancer fucking sucks*. No one should ever be so presumptuous as to tell us it is some sort of gift or life lesson or divine plan.

When people interject their religious faith into our cancer story

Privately praying for us?
Great! And thank you so much!
Quoting scripture to us? Telling us God controls all and insinuating that He delivered cancer to Shelley because He's testing us? Preaching that He has a plan that includes her predestined outcome regardless of her treatment?
Oh, my goodness, *please* don't.
I have a subsection in a couple of pages on why people shouldn't opine on how someone's cancer occurred. Sadly, the very few comments to us implying it was God's will that gave Shelley cancer were just the worst of the worst.
Indeed, I'm probably the last person in the world qualified to lecture anyone about religion. But that also means I don't want to be lectured, either. I've always felt that one's religious beliefs should be categorically personal. It's how I hold my own. Though this will never happen, I wish we all could somehow come to terms with the fact that spiritual perceptions differ, and that doesn't make them any less valid.

Before broaching the religious topic to a family in a cancer fight, again, *one needs to know the audience*. Those with strong religious faith and those who are atheists (or, perhaps, anything in between) often deny the plausibility of one another's staunch beliefs and convictions. If they do, an ensuing, unhelpful step can occur if they proceed to engage in unwinnable arguments attempting to tread on opposing views for the purpose of "correcting" the other's religious disagreement.

In determining these parameters of a conversation between friend and cancer fighter, an easy, productive rule to follow is that – no matter *what* one believes – the cancer fighter's spiritual perceptions prevail at that moment. *Always.* I think it's best for others to avoid religious ("God is watching over you") or atheistic ("Cancer is proof that God doesn't exist") framing of someone else's diagnosis altogether. Or at least until it is unmistakably known what the patient's convictions are.

For outwardly religious survivors and their families, spiritual conversations can be appropriate and quite beneficial. One of my colleagues sadly lost her husband after a long battle with cancer. She is a very religious individual, and her faith brought her great comfort during the most terrible time in her life.

But this doesn't work for those who don't share that faith, regardless of whether you may think "it's for their own good." And the assumption that we all (should) possess similar religious views could cause more unnecessary emotional harm. As I wrote earlier, my family's cancer story isn't available for framing by anyone other than us.

From the start, we made it clear on our CaringBridge site that we were not open to assertions that cancer is part of God's plan, and that He's watching over us (but for some reason gave Shelley cancer anyway). However, a limited few refused to hear that message and felt license to impose their views. As well intentioned as it always was, it didn't help. We perceived their religious declarations to be little but flippantly, if not defiantly, disconnected responses to our painful cancer realities.

If friends and colleagues believe that prayer will help, then, by all means, I hope they pray. They can pray for the cancer fighter's strength, the surgeon's skills, or for treatment effectiveness among other things. I would never assert that it doesn't help, because it very well might. But, again, outwardly and boldly asserting that God controls all may cause some patients and caregivers to see upsetting and counterproductive logical flaws.

The best thing to do is to follow the survivor's lead on this. If the patient and family members are openly religious while discussing their cancer, it's probably safe to engage on that level. If they don't bring religion up, however, you really shouldn't, either. If, for whatever reason, you do anyway, I hope you won't take it personally when you're asked to avoid defining their situation by your beliefs.

Just leave it to the survivor and family members to frame their experience as they see fit. Because, like it or not, your approval or disapproval with how they do so is completely irrelevant to them. Until you ascertain where the boundaries lie, my best advice is to avoid religious or atheistic description of someone else's cancer fight. And once you do figure them out, everyone will be best served if you stay well within those boundaries.

When people comment on why the cancer occurred

Heather M., our good friend who began her fight with breast cancer seven years before Shelley's battle commenced, was diagnosed in late spring. As a result, her chemo-induced hair loss took place during the seasonal heat and humidity of a Missouri summer. Therefore, she decided to forgo the use of a wig. She was not the least bit embarrassed about going out in public with a perfectly bald head. (Nor should she have been!)

One day, she and her baby boy were in the checkout line at a grocery store when a middle-aged man looked at her head and stoically asked, "So what did you do?"

Perplexed, Heather responded, "I'm sorry, but I don't understand what you're asking me."

"Well, you're bald, so I assume you have cancer," he said without embarrassment or hesitation. "What did you do to get cancer?" Heather was completely taken aback by his audacity. Clearly, this man, with classlessness and apathy on full display (and no mouth-filter within earshot), was probably interested in avoiding all cancer risk factors. That's understandable. But he did so at Heather's emotional expense, and he committed two social blunders in the process. First, it was almost as if he assumed Heather's medical life was his business. And, second, he explicitly blamed a cancer fighter for her cancer. Enormously bad form on both counts, indeed.

The American Cancer Society states that one in eight women will get breast cancer.[32] Does the "why" *truly* matter to the point that someone, somehow, feels the need to weigh in about it? As is the situation for all cancer fighters, Heather's cancer simply was what it was. She'd always lived a healthy lifestyle. She regularly exercised, she ate healthy foods, and she never smoked. Risk factors are only that: factors containing statistical consistency. But they don't always hold true.

For example, though we obviously decrease our chances of getting lung cancer (and various other cancers), heart disease, and COPD by not smoking, there are no guarantees. Dana Reeve (widow of *Superman* actor, Christopher Reeve) died of lung cancer at the age of 44, though she never smoked.[33] On the other hand, my grandfather smoked during much of his adult life but lived until he was 88 when he essentially died of old age. Clearly these occurrences were somewhat anomalous, but they do happen on occasion.

Why some people get cancer and others with similar lifestyles don't is generally a biological mystery. It probably has more to do with bad luck than anything else. Going so far as to suggest a "justification" ("You shouldn't have used birth control pills," "You shouldn't have eaten so much meat," "You shouldn't have used hair color," "You shouldn't have smoked when you were younger," etc.) isn't a productive conversation in the least. It will only make patients feel guilty and subsequently even worse than they already do. What would criticizing them accomplish other than implying that the patient somehow deserved to get cancer? My belief is that the subject should be avoided altogether.

Dealing with those who push unsolicited medical advice

As I've stated many times, our friends and colleagues care a great deal about us and have the best of intentions. But a few of them didn't always seem to understand that it's the job of our board-certified oncology physicians to keep up to date on breakthroughs and advancements in detection and treatment. And that's precisely what they do.

It's very common to read articles in the newspaper or see a network television newsmagazine about new cancer research. Internet videos can provide such information as well. As a result of doing so, a few of our acquaintances seemed to become, more or less, self-anointed cancer "experts" who eagerly wished to share what they saw as meaningful information or research updates they assumed we and our oncology team didn't know about. Again, we were fully aware that they were only trying to help us in every way they could. Our normal response was a general thank-you, and then we'd change the subject of the conversation.

What some people may not realize is that, very likely, patients and caregivers (like Shelley and me) already know far more than most others outside of the medical community regarding their own cancer and how best to treat and cope with it. And that's because of their repeated interactions with oncologists and nurses during numerous appointment consultations.

Other acquaintances, however, advanced our discomfort level much further by trying to convince us about internet misinformation, which advocated the use of completely unproven (and, I would surmise, useless) alternative therapies.

There is no question that cases of what is called "spontaneous remission" have been documented. It takes place when one's cancer somehow regresses or even disappears without treatment or when conventional treatments appear not to have succeeded. Some instances are indeed scientifically unexplainable at this point. But evidence of this phenomenon is anecdotal at best, and true occurrences are extremely rare.[34]

Those few who are lucky enough to actually experience a spontaneous remission may even attribute it to a perceived stimulus or alternative therapy such as prayer or consumption of certain herbs, supplements, or other dietary changes. And, of course, this initially looks attractive since *no one* wants to sustain the terrible side effects of chemo. However, it's always important to be more than a little suspicious if it sounds too good to be true. There just isn't any solid, empirical evidence to remotely substantiate such cause-effect claims. As one noted oncologist very diplomatically put it, perhaps there really are miracle treatments or cures yet to be discovered that could completely change the course of cancer care. But, he continued, when it comes to alternative therapies, "history suggests to us that we have to be skeptics here. If it was so simple then [cancer] would have been solved a long time ago."[35]

Shelley and I didn't think twice about following through with the wisdom of conventional therapy. In fact, use of anything but modern medicine never occurred to us. We had every reason to trust the statistical probabilities of science and, therefore, put our faith into the hands of our capable oncology team without hesitation. To us, it was a proverbial "no brainer" decision and one we never regretted for a moment.

However, in spite of my repeated polite attempts at changing the subject, one of our friends was taking no hints, and she was quite insistent in attempting to advance her alternative therapy ideas. It finally got to the point where I felt I had no other recourse but to hold up my hand and say, with exasperation, "Please stop. Please. Just. Stop. I appreciate your caring. I know you mean well. But you're not an oncologist or any other type of physician. Hopefully, you'll never get cancer. If you do, you can determine your own course of treatment as you see fit. Shelley and I are going to stick with evidence-based science." Of course, that didn't change her mind, but it finally got her to stop talking about it.

"You need a better attitude"

As I was leaving a store one afternoon, I ran into an acquaintance I hadn't seen in years (who, thankfully, had no family cancer experience). When I disclosed Shelley's ongoing battle, I guess she must have thought my demeanor sounded a bit depressed. Much to my surprise, she proceeded to lecture me about my ostensibly negative approach at that moment. "Keith, you need a better attitude than that, and so does Shelley," she said. She was basing her entire assessment of our "need" for an improved mindset exclusively on the 60–90 seconds I spent explaining to her what was happening with Shelley.

Now on the surface, of course there's nothing wrong with promoting a good attitude. Shelley and I always did our best on that front. But repetitively hearing it from others can be overly simplistic and quite patronizing to a veteran cancer fighter (and even to her caregiver) whose treatment side effects were cumulatively worsening. And since we were seven months into treatment at the time, it wasn't exactly the first occasion someone had commented to us on the virtues of a good attitude.

However, my acquaintance emphatically persisted and did so while literally shaking her finger at me. "Keith, go home and tell your wife that, now. My friend with cancer had a good attitude, and *that's* why she's alive today." I imagine the acquaintance felt she was enlightening me with some sort of groundbreaking, revolutionary cancer development. Though she *obviously* meant well, she didn't proactively think about how and what she was communicating in presuming we had a poor attitude, which was something that wasn't even true in the first place. I did my best, during this unnecessary and unwanted sermon, to suppress my burgeoning displeasure.

Perhaps I was just growing weary of some repeated comments over the months that, no matter how we were feeling, Shelley and I should always maintain a positive mental approach. Or, maybe, in conducting my own novice cancer research, I simply knew better. But it's almost become an age-old question: *Why did some people without any medical training and no experience in fighting cancer or in caregiving veer outside of their lanes by practically insisting they had answers that we and our oncology team did not?*

A highly informative and heart-rending book I read about cancer was *The Emperor of All Maladies: A Biography of Cancer* by renowned oncologist Dr. Siddhartha Mukherjee. In an interview about his published work, Dr. Mukherjee was asked if a positive mental attitude was a true difference-maker in whether or not someone would beat cancer. His response was a reserved, but succinct and emphatic *no*. "A positive attitude does not cure cancer, any more than a negative one causes it," he said.[36] He further outlined damaging psychological effects that may result when someone pushes a better outlook as the key to a cure:

"I think it does a nasty disservice to patients. A woman with breast cancer already has her plate full, and you want to go and tell her that 'the reason you're not getting better is because you're not thinking positively'? Put yourself in that woman's position and think what it feels like to be told 'your attitude is to blame for why you're not getting better.' I think it's nasty."[37]

Amen to that.

For the record, I've never seen anyone cope with cancer in a more positive way than my wife, even in spite of a number of critical setbacks. Equally, for the record (as Dr. Mukherjee concurred), a good attitude may indeed help the cancer fighter keep up the resolve in tolerating the terrible, continuous side effects of treatment – treatment that may *or* may not be effectively working. In and of itself, however, attitude *doesn't* kill or eradicate cancer cells.

In my growing impatience and frustration with my acquaintance's cancer portrayal, all I wanted was to end the conversation and get back home with my store items. Instead, however, I decided to offer her a little gift of knowledge. And a ration of harsh reality.

To the best of my ability, I tried to calmly and graciously explain why she shouldn't talk that way to anyone in a cancer family, even though she meant well. I provided her with some perspective so that she might empathize a little more with people who were facing something she couldn't fully grasp without experiencing it firsthand.

I told her it's important for her to understand that many patients with very early detected, considerably localized, or less aggressive cancers have a good chance to completely beat the disease, and that their outlook or attitude would play little, if any, role in the process.

But my father, for example, who was diagnosed with an inoperable stage IV cancer, essentially received a death-sentence the moment he learned he had the disease. Dad's passing, after nearly six and a half years of absolutely willing himself through grueling, horrific, and, ultimately, ineffective treatment, had *nothing* to do with his attitude, toughness, or ability to fight. To suggest otherwise would be insulting. He died for one reason *only*: because medical research had not advanced enough at that time to provide treatment that could cure him or prolong his life.

"Look, I *know* it's not your intent," I concluded, "but when you tell us we need a better attitude, it almost sounds like you're blaming us for Shelley going through a rough patch with her treatment. And that's not cool."

As I spoke, my friend's facial expression completely changed, and her eyes teared up a bit. "Oh my God, I was just trying to help, and I only made things worse," she responded, in what seemed to be a defining moment of self-realization. I put my arm around her and assured her that her good intentions spoke much louder than her words. She wished me well, and we went our separate ways.

"If you're not getting better, you need to go to a different clinic"

During the arduous journey of treatment, it is common for patients to experience setbacks. It *doesn't* mean the cancer institute isn't doing its job or that it has less access to cutting edge treatments. Everyone's disease is different. Hence, sadly, regardless of treatment, not everyone beats cancer. Therefore, a patient's temporary stumbling block should never be seen as an invitation to outwardly push the idea that there should be a change in physicians, venue, or treatment regimen. That is for the cancer fighters to decide on their own in consultation with their oncology teams.

As I stated earlier, this was the case with one of my wife's friends. Again, the friend's message was obviously well intended, but its content was pointless and without merit. We go to a regionally prominent cancer center with multiple-award-winning, board-certified oncologists and oncology nurses. And the reason is to have access to the best and most successful treatments known to humankind. No one should make us feel obligated to spend precious time and energy needlessly justifying our well-informed decisions and treatment plans.

I've spent a lot of time in this chapter explaining what we didn't want our friends and co-workers to say to us. But if you're wondering what *should* be said in general to cancer fighters and their caregivers amid all the potential differences of perception and interpretation, it can actually be pretty simple.

Don't try to apply the Golden Rule by talking to them the way you *think* you'd want to be addressed if the roles were reversed. Because, unless you've been there, you truly don't know. At the end of the day, whatever you say to them should be for their benefit, not to make yourself feel better.

Simply share the human experience of co-grieving with them. Offer empathy, compassion, support, and any help they may need or that they ask for. If their lawn needs to be mowed, mow it for them. If they want you to be upbeat, be upbeat. If they request your avoiding the topic of their cancer to provide them with a temporary escape at that moment, talk about something else. If they wish for you to pray with them, do so. *If they just need to hear someone else say how unfair life has been to them, say it.*

And if the right words seem elusive? Try the simple act of listening. Let them vent about the rigors and physical horrors of treatment or the stress and demands of caregiving *without* commentary or opinions on how you think they should be handling it. Psychologically, it will be, more than likely, *precisely* what they need.

CHAPTER 12

Radiation Is Quick, Repetitive, and to the Point

When radium was discovered, no one knew that it would prove useful in hospitals. The work was one of pure science. And this is a proof that scientific work must not be considered [only] from the point of view of the direct usefulness of it.
-Marie Curie, discoverer of radium and polonium

Like all cancer treatments, the whys and hows of radiation are complex, and it can be used at a variety of times during the treatment regimen. For Shelley it was conducted post-lumpectomy. Since a lumpectomy specifically removes the tumor and closely surrounding breast tissue, radiation targets a wider breast area to kill any potentially remaining cancer cells, thereby reducing the chance of future recurrences.[38] Shelley's routine, beginning in mid-July, would be 30 rounds – Monday through Friday for six weeks.

We were told that radiation's side effects are normally fairly minimal, although there can be exceptions of course. And like other cancer treatments, the side effects accumulate and are a little more noticeable in the latter stages of the schedule.

But prior to the start of this new treatment, Shelley needed to undergo rather extensive post-surgical physical therapy. The surgery notably stiffened and limited the range of motion in her side and shoulder. Radiation therapy would require Shelley's ability to put her hand *well* above her head so that the targeted breast tissue was easily reached, which was something she couldn't do in the least prior to PT. She needed significantly more flexibility with her shoulder and latissimus dorsi muscle. Since she had considerable post-surgical pain and limited movement, re-strengthening the area was also necessary. Stretching exercises and working out with lighter weights became a part of the at-home routine when she wasn't in the PT clinic.

According to breastcancer.org, careful planning, also known as "mapping," is necessary before radiation treatment can commence.[39] This planning helps ensure highly specific targeting and the full benefit of radiation with minimal impact on other parts of the body. Thankfully, Shelley quickly made significant progress in regaining both strength and flexibility. In the span of just a week, she went from having little movement in her shoulder area to being able to position her arm high enough to undergo the radiation planning and mapping procedure.

Of course, one of the great myths of radiation treatment is that the patient might be "radioactive" and therefore dangerous to surrounding people for a time after each round. Rest assured, it's not true at all. Each dose is delivered instantly and precisely with no residual effect.[40] But that certainly didn't stop us from occasionally joking about it with one another. After one of her early treatments, Shelley came back to the waiting room with a big grin and said to me, "Does it look like I have a special 'glow' about me?" "Yes," I responded with wide-eyed, exaggerated agreement, "and your smile almost seems new, and cle-ar." A woman sitting within earshot apparently appreciated both puns. "Oh, gawd, that's terrible," she outwardly chuckled. "And I'm gonna say the same things to my husband when he comes out from his treatment."

Throughout the six weeks, we found radiation to be pretty much what we were told it would be: quick and relatively painless. Moderate fatigue and redness/soreness in the treated areas were Shelley's main, but slow-developing, reactions. By the time her regimen was done, she experienced noticeable breast soreness, and she looked (and felt) as if she had a *terrible* sunburn on her upper right side and breast area.

Shelley's final radiation round took place on Tuesday, August 21. To commemorate, we had our picture taken together while holding her completion-of-radiation certificate from Missouri Cancer Associates. But there wasn't any of the euphoria attached to it that we had on May 4 when she'd finished chemotherapy, back when we had realistic hope that the end of radiation would be the conclusion of all cancer treatment. In fact, this ritual almost seemed a bit depressing, knowing that she had so much more to go with the chemotherapy pill over the following six months.

Nonetheless, we still recognized it as the milestone it was, and we had planned a private, discreet moment of reserved "celebration" – dinner alone together at a local restaurant, which was how we wanted it to be. At the last minute, however, word of those plans got out, and dinner somehow quickly and spontaneously morphed into five other people joining us. At the outset, Shelley and I were a tad uncomfortable with this larger impromptu gathering. But we also recognized that such a get-together did seem to mean a lot to the others. No question that the seven of us celebrated a little more than Shelley and I would have alone. It was a nice, temporary escape. But when we returned home later in the evening, we wept for a bit at what might have been.

Shelley started her oral chemo regimen of Xeloda® (capecitabine) on August 25. If she could tolerate its potency, she would take eight pills daily for two weeks, have one week off, then repeat the cycle for the next six months. As with all chemo treatments, there could be strong side effects such as diarrhea, nausea, mouth and throat sores, dehydration, and damaging dryness and irritation on the palms of her hands and bottoms of her feet among many others.[41] We hoped they wouldn't be intolerable, but we had to wait and see.

As we would begin yet another method of treatment, we again feared the unknown magnitude of new future side effects. And since the original chemo didn't quite get everything, even more long-term prognosis fears pervaded our emotions. Would completion of this fourth therapy segment finally get her to remission? Or were we instead running out of options? This woman had endured repeated violations of her body over the previous eight months. At this point, she was so tired of everything, and all she wanted was time to let herself heal. Unfortunately, that process wouldn't even begin for at least *another* six months.

CHAPTER 13

Autumn and Cancer

Life starts all over again when it gets crisp in the fall...
-F. Scott Fitzgerald

As we headed into autumn, our cancer fight had taken us through the entirety of the 2018 winter, spring, and summer seasons. September arrived, and we were still learning about the side effects of Shelley's new chemo pill routine and how to cope with them. We hoped that the change to cooler weather would somehow be of some benefit to her. Aside from the cancer, autumn is just a beautiful time of year. If late-August and early-September social media posts are any indicator, there are probably millions of people across the country who have a serious love affair with autumn. And Shelley and I are right there with them.

Though seasonal changes aren't quite as distinct in Southern California as in much of the U.S., I still enjoyed fall celebrations while growing up near Los Angeles in the 1960s. Halloween, my birthday, and Thanksgiving take place in a span of three to four weeks each year. My childhood autumn memories are chock-full of trick-or-treating, birthday parties, and a long, celebratory November week-end of family, football, and great food. When a two-week Christmas-vacation hiatus from grade school occurred a month or so later, the year would end on a high note. Therefore, October, November, and December have always been my favorite months.

There's indeed something magical about autumn. When I left California right after I finished grad school and a new job led me to Northeast Iowa (where Shelley was born and raised), I noticed how the Midwest's seasonal changes were amplified beyond my wildest imagination. In that part of the country, autumn signifies that the long, hot, oppressively humid dog days of summer have *finally* reached an end. The fall harvest begins. Daylight hours are shorter. Wardrobes change from shorts and tank tops to blue jeans and sweatshirts as there's an inviting chill in the air. Decorations and inventory in stores of all kinds come to reflect the seasonal transformations. I love the slow emergence of autumn foliage that begins in late September or early October. It beautifully complements the pumpkins and cornstalks that adorn neighborhood porches. For several weeks in October and November, the wind gently blows through the colorful trees, and bright scarlet, yellow, and orange leaves almost seem to dance in festivity. It's a season that cries out for celebration.

On a cool, overcast October Saturday afternoon in the late 1990s, Shelley and I unknowingly began a tradition of hosting an annual get-together we now call the pumpkin party. Along with our two small children, Shelley and I dressed in jeans and hoodies to match the seasonal temperatures. A few friends and their young kids joined us in driving to a local pumpkin farm in rural mid-Missouri to pick pumpkins. We then caravanned back to our house to enjoy pizza, apple cider, and pumpkin cookies while we watched college football on TV. Since then, we've had these gatherings each October. Time has passed, all of our kids have grown and moved away, but, decades later, the annual party has increased in guest numbers, and it still includes the original parents. It's our way every year of officially welcoming fall.

As September 2018 concluded, our house was slowly, but surely, filling with autumn and Halloween decorations. And soon, Shelley and I would continue another of our annual family traditions by popping some popcorn, turning out all the lights, and spending a couple of hours on a Friday or Saturday night watching our favorite Halloween movie, *Hocus Pocus*.

That year, the personal significance of October marking Breast Cancer Awareness Month was definitely not lost on us. With cancer in the equation, this particular autumn obviously would be unique from those in the past. Nonetheless, we hoped the season would provide a temporary but welcome escape from our oncology concerns.

Saturday, September 29, was one of our first days of true fall weather in mid-Missouri with morning temperatures dipping into the mid to upper 40s. Shelley and I threw on a fleece jacket and hoodie and went downtown to our favorite coffee house for a bagel and a pumpkin spice latte. It was a warm and tasty beginning to a crisp autumn morning. We then headed to a local farm and garden center to get some more home decorations for fall – chrysanthemums, gourds, and pumpkins.

There were large barns packed with pumpkins of all shapes and sizes. There were so many pumpkins it looked like a genuine sea of orange. The farm even sold pink pumpkins to match October's breast cancer theme with the sale proceeds going to breast cancer research. We purchased the brightest pink one. In addition, we also bought two medium-large carving pumpkins, a variety of gourds with multiple shapes and colors, and even some dried corn for home decoration. It was such amazing autumn fun!

In the early afternoon, we made our way to a local winery for a glass of cabernet. We chowed down on sandwiches we had brought with us and enjoyed the beautiful, relaxing lake and meadow scenery. It was a really nice day in so many ways, but cancer and its treatment refused to let us completely escape its vise-like grip. By midafternoon, Shelley was exhausted, so we drove home, where she promptly took a two-hour nap. Her energy level had clearly taken a recent tumble with her new treatment.

Besides fatigue, it didn't take long for the Xeloda regimen to affect

Shelley in other ways. It created a lot of discomfort in her hands and feet. Her palms and bottoms of her feet were developing redness, irritation, and blisters. Walking any sort of distance had started to become an issue for her.

With the calendar turning to October, we were only five weeks into the new six-month, eight-daily-pills plan when even more physical problems started to transpire. By the following weekend, something was clearly wrong. Shelley had no energy along with other accompanying internal issues including dull abdominal pain. On Monday, October 8, she was almost unable to get out of bed, let alone go in to work. She was feeling so bad that we went in to Missouri Cancer Associates, where she was given a liter of intravenous (IV) fluids in the infusion area. Again, one of the notable side effects of Xeloda is dehydration. Those who are on this medication must take proper steps to stay hydrated, even if they don't feel thirsty. And Shelley would be the first to confess she hadn't done very well on that front.

After receiving the fluids, Shelley immediately felt much better, so I took her home and then went over to campus to teach my class. But by the time I returned, she had regressed. The following morning, she felt even worse, so we returned to MCA, again, for more IV fluids. During this time, Dr. Makarian stopped by to visit, followed by a couple of our nurses. Each of them asked Shelley if she had been drinking extra fluids and taking other meds to combat her side effects. Shelley's answer was a rather meek, "Well, no, not really." As if on cue, each of them asked, eyes wide open and loudly, "Well, why not?"

Their eye contact – quite perturbed eye contact – was directed at *me*, as if it were my fault that Shelley didn't consume the electrolyte beverages, glasses of water, and side-effect pills I constantly placed in front of her and had pleaded with her to drink and take. And when I made it abundantly clear to everyone (while giggling) that I indeed pushed the fluids and meds, the fire was redirected toward Shelley. I admit that it was a rather enjoyable, however momentary, experience.

"You need to listen to your husband!" Dr. Makarian exclaimed.

One of the nurses added, "He's a good man who's taking good care of you. Do what he says!"

Ah, nirvana. And vindication.

Shelley reacted to the symptoms. I, instead, wanted to be proactive, to head symptoms off at the pass, so to speak, before they started. As I've repeatedly told my students over the years, "fire prevention is a lot easier than firefighting." But who knew I possessed such wisdom?

We continued the IV fluids for five straight days, and Dr. Makarian said we'd be suspending the Xeloda for a week in the hope that Shelley's insides would recalibrate, reboot, and recover. It was a good call, and there was noticeable improvement in the way she soon felt.

For obvious reasons, Shelley and I discussed the idea of canceling the pumpkin party we'd scheduled for the next weekend, and I gave her full veto power. In the end, she said, "It's the most fun autumn thing we do every year. It's tradition. How can we *not* have the pumpkin party?"

Shelley slowly continued to improve, and the party was on. Our friends and colleagues arrived with autumn-themed snacks to complement the seasonal ambience. It was a really nice get-together that began with an exciting fourth quarter of a college football game on TV. After our pizza dinner, we all moved outside to the patio. The weather was a bit chilly under the dark October sky, so we brought out blankets and sat near a warm fire in the fire pit. We drank hot cider and sampled a variety of pumpkin beers, and we finished the evening by roasting marshmallows and making tasty s'mores. Shelley's perpetual smile throughout the festivities was indicative of the party's obvious success. Overall, the distraction of these autumn activities couldn't have come at a better time for us with Shelley having felt perhaps her worst since the Adriamycin/Cytoxan treatments earlier in the year.

CHAPTER 14

Perfect

Don't wait for the perfect moment, take the moment and make it perfect.

-Zoey Sayward

Wednesday, November 14, was a good day for Shelley. In fact, one might argue that it was perfect. Since we hadn't had all that many of them during the past 11 months, we really wanted to make note of and celebrate the ones we got.

As consequence of that awful early October week when she felt so terrible, Shelley had to postpone her planned, mom/daughter daytrip to Kansas City to find her perfect dress for Karen's upcoming spring wedding. This was devastating for Shelley. (And for Karen. And me.) But on this cold mid-November day, she was able to redeem her rain check for the outing in KC. That morning the sun had finally come out after a couple of snowy, dreary days.

Shelley's alarm went off at 5:30 am, and the song waking her up was perfect. I literally meant that it was "Perfect," a tune by Ed Sheeran that Shelley believes perfectly describes Karen's and Jake's relationship together.

At about 7:00, she got into her car and drove to Kansas City for her adventure with Karen.

The two of them had a perfectly good time. They enjoyed a filling lunch at a barbeque place in KC, and then headed out to shop in search of Shelley's wedding attire. And, bingo, she found the ideal dress! Afterward, they stopped at a coffee house to warm up with a hot drink on a very chilly day. How fitting that "Perfect" came on the radio for Shelley to hear again on her drive back to Columbia.

During the previous weeks, Shelley had become far more diligent about drinking more daily fluids and taking her medications to diminish the side effects of her chemotherapy pill. In addition, the oncologist dialed back the Xeloda dosage by 25% after starting at the maximum. Shelley was now down to six daily pills from the previous eight, but she felt much better as a result. Not pre-cancer-better of course. Not even close. The chemo in pill form – by any measure – was still quite uncomfortable. But, comparatively speaking, she was having better days, and having them a little more often.

Three weeks later, December 6, 2018 marked a year to the day since diagnosis. Over the course of that year, Shelley withstood 16 rounds of chemotherapy, three surgeries, 30 rounds of radiation, and about three months (of the scheduled six) of oral chemotherapy. It had often been hell up to that point, and we still weren't done.

As fate would have it, Shelley's first post-radiation mammogram was scheduled on that one-year anniversary, and she viewed the timing with a little angst. But I countered that it was actually the best day for it to take place; that we had to start perceiving December 6 not with negativity, but as a mark of survivorship. Of course, the scheduled mammogram had been on our radar for a couple of months. And our nervous anticipation intensified as the date neared. Would there be more bad news? Or would there be an all clear?

The day started very positively. Early in the morning, my niece and her husband welcomed their first child, and my brother and sister-in-law became first-time grandparents. We'd hoped that was some sort of good omen. After the mammogram took place, we sat and waited for a while in the examination room until our surgeon, Dr. Peterson, walked in to announce the results.

"Your mammogram looks clear and gorgeous," she said. I threw my fists upward in victory. Shelley could only weep in relief. It was indeed another *perfect* day.

We had long since come to the point of never taking anything for granted, and it should be noted that Shelley's mammogram the previous year did not pick up the tumor. She has very dense breast tissue, which makes it difficult to detect abnormalities. But we took the good news for what it was that December 6 day: *good news*. And we knew of the future, and necessary vigilance that would need to take place. She'd be scanned every six months alternating MRIs with mammograms and numerous checkups in between. It's a small price to pay to keep my perfect wife with me.

CHAPTER 15

The Shadow of Trepidation

We cannot selectively numb emotions. When we numb the painful emotions, we also numb the positive emotions.

-Brené Brown

On New Year's Eve, Mark, one of my good friends and an especially supportive one throughout Shelley's cancer treatment, texted me a meme that appropriately said, *"Fuck 2018! Bring on 2019!"* That pretty much summed up my end-of-year feelings. In fact, those words were the entirety of my private, midnight champagne toast to Shelley. "Hear, hear," she responded with emphasis and agreement, as we drank our half-filled flutes of bubbly.

By the start of the New Year, Shelley's treatment was very near its conclusion. She had only about six weeks remaining of her oral chemotherapy. But the snowballing side-effect issues with her hands and feet were becoming less tolerable by the day. In mid-January, Dr. Makarian reluctantly cut Shelley's daily pill intake by one, from six to five. Not long afterward, it had to be reduced to four. The side effects were just too powerful. We hoped this would make things more manageable until completion. On the other hand, of course, we wanted the dose level, which had already been reduced by 25% back in October, to do everything the drug was designed to do. And that was to kill every last, individual cancer cell her original chemo left behind the previous spring. It was an anxious balancing act between eliminating all the cancer while not being overwhelmed by the side effects. I will admit that lessening the dose worried me, considerably.

Shelley officially completed her primary cancer treatment at 6:48 pm on the evening of February 17, 2019. Having taken her final chemotherapy pill of a six-month regimen, it was exactly 438 excruciating days after she was diagnosed. February 18 was the first day of her long awaited healing process. We knew it would take many months, if not years, of recovery to undo all the physical and nerve damage, assuming her battered body could make it all the way back to how it was before the ordeal began. As of this 2020 writing, she will continue for the foreseeable future with adjuvant hormonal medications such as tamoxifen, letrozole, and Ibrance® (palbociclib) to help ward off the development of secondary or returning tumors.

Throughout the 14 months of her treatment, it was a prospective day we had envisioned with hope and anticipation. I'd assumed we'd both feel immediate joy in that the burden would finally be lifted from our shoulders. But when treatment was actually completed, neither Shelley nor I felt as if we'd won much of anything. There was no exclamation of "We beat it!" Perhaps that was because our balloon of hope was so loudly popped the previous June, after we had let our guard down and believed a complete cure was on the near horizon. I was still haunted by the false elation I'd felt back then and the temporary crash of anguish and hopelessness that followed soon after.

On treatment-finale night, we felt tired. We felt numb. We felt the lingering fear of wondering if this would ever be completely over; if the six weeks of radiation and six months of daily chemo pills had completed the job. Other than the passage of extended time, how could we possibly know?

Nonetheless, the conclusion of treatment was, by far, the biggest of our cancer milestones, and one that could neither be ignored nor even discounted. And we *did* celebrate. A group of my closest colleagues joined us for dinner at one of our favorite Mexican restaurants.

Afterward, we all returned to our house where we shared a bottle of champagne Shelley and I had been saving for this special day.

But while we were definitely glad it was over, we still approached the marker with uncertainty. Aside from the obvious long-term physical road to recovery that Shelley had ahead of her, we both experienced a tremendous amount of uneasiness and fear about what was to come. Apparently, this is common. According to oncology social worker, Dr. Jill Mitchell, there are genuine reasons to feel this type of post-treatment anxiety.[42] Three of them in particular stand out for us:

- *Fear of recurrence* – I suspect both Shelley and I will experience into perpetuity a great deal of uneasiness and apprehension when a scheduled mammogram or MRI nears. These state-of-the-art imagery tests detect the visuals of tumors but not individual cancer cells. If just one cell survived all the chemo and radiation, it wouldn't be picked up by any test, and it very well could one day materialize as another malignant tumor.

- *Lingering side effects* – Once her regular chemo treatment was completed, Shelley's hair very slowly began to return. But, months later, some of her side effects have yet to even begin subsiding. Pain and neuropathy in her feet still make walking very difficult. The same issues in her hands cause dexterity problems when much of her professional work involves meticulous computer use. Though it's getting better, she also cites chemo brain as something that continues to cause occasional memory lapses. The removal of so many lymph nodes drastically increases her chances of developing lymphedema, a malady that can cause skin and bacterial infections and other annoying symptoms. Shelley outwardly wonders if any of these side effects will ever completely heal.

- *Going from daily, weekly, or monthly doctor's visits to only once every several months* – While multiple appointments throughout treatment certainly taxed our professional and personal time, there was a firm level of comfort in seeing medical experts on a routine basis. They could quickly assess and immediately attempt to correct any physical problems we encountered. Now we must determine for ourselves what physical changes and potential symptoms merit alerting her physician beyond the new infrequent appointment schedule.

Of course, there is the very realistic possibility that Shelley became cancer-free. Since what was left of the tumor had been removed, the subsequent six weeks of radiation and the six months of oral chemo may very well have succeeded in eradicating whatever cancer was left. But, as is the case with life in general, there are no guarantees. So we wait. Shelley and her oncology team will have to be vigilant for years to come.

Our ability to completely exhale from this horror story may never materialize. Even in post-treatment, Shelley's past cancer is a shadow of trepidation that will undoubtedly linger over us for the rest of our lives. The research of Sophia Smith, associate professor at the Duke University School of Nursing, corroborates this. She indicates that many survivors actually develop PTSD *after* cancer treatment has concluded.[43]

Added to one's emotional stress could be an inability to pay for these early detection, post-treatment tests, which are needed to keep an eagle eye on prospective recurrence. Obviously, cancer is more likely to return to someone who's already had it. Therefore, a post-cancer narrative could never be complete without including a commentary of periodic issues stemming from our country's private, profit-based health insurance.

Good healthcare plans and medical access are crucial to not only beating cancer but for keeping it away once you've had it. But even good plans can still have prohibitive deductibles of $5,000 or more. For lower- or middle-class income families (we are the latter), it can wreak havoc on financial well-being. In fact, one in eight cancer patients in the U.S. must refuse treatment because they simply can't afford it.[44] For a country as rich as ours, this is unconscionable.

Throughout her professional life, Shelley dutifully paid her monthly insurance premiums by way of her employer's health plan. The insurance company gladly accepted her payments while she was pre-cancer healthy, when she rarely needed to use their services beyond routine checkups. And, obviously, she kept up with monthly payments throughout her treatment and after it concluded. I think it's reasonable to think that those of us who are lucky enough to have health insurance should be able – at *all* times – to count on the coverage we've paid for when a life-threatening issue such as cancer comes up. After all, we always held up *our* end of the bargain.

But then in addition to our already existing cancer woes, our company sometimes decided not to cover a test or procedure recommended as necessary by our oncologist. It's what I refer to as the insurance company playing the "asshole card." The company's verdict, of course, is based exclusively on exceptionally wealthy executives' financial decisions *instead of the patient's legitimate medical needs*. In other words, a multibillion dollar corporation arbitrarily decides to deny coverage for, say, a $5,000 claim that objective medical and scientific experts have deemed necessary for appropriate treatment. Or for early detection of a potential recurring cancer after it's gone into remission or is "arrested."

Coupled with the deductible, this now translates to $10,000 or more out of pocket for the person insured, and that doesn't even include the cost of monthly premiums. It's bad enough having to cope with cancer. But when our ostensible insurance ally turned on us financially during the process, it exacerbated everything. I will say that our post-deductible coverage occurred *far* more often than not. But all it takes is one time to be a tremendous financial and emotional burden. And that naturally includes worrying about when it might arbitrarily happen again. *Because it will*. And, of course, that $5,000 isn't even a fraction of a single drop of water in an Olympic-sized swimming pool to the insurance company. But it may be two months of net income that could be critical for the patient's financial survival.

This most recently happened to us when our insurance refused to pre-certify a standard, post-treatment, and *necessary* MRI. As a result, the scheduled test was delayed. Years of patient coverage for such follow-up MRIs has long been the norm for cancer treatment and for the insurance industry. And since our company would be on the hook for an advanced return of Shelley's cancer, *it could actually save them money in the long run to fund this scan* by catching it early. It's a perfect example of English Scholar Robert Burton's warning of *penny wise, pound foolish*[45] and it represents everything that is wrong with for-profit healthcare insurance companies in the U.S. The harsh reality is that they care far more about their financial bottom line than they do about any of the people they're supposed to serve.

When this dispute to cover the MRI occurred, Shelley and I took immediate action. If insurance companies initially deny you coverage, they're hoping you quickly give up, quietly accept their unjust verdict, and pay for a claim or procedure yourself (or simply forgo the procedure). If you're in that situation, *don't give up without giving them an aggressively protracted fight*. We didn't accept it, and we decided to pester them. We repeatedly contacted our insurance with unrelenting persistence. Then we tightened the screws even more by asking our oncologist to get involved in a peer-to-peer conference with a physician within the insurance company.

Apparently, Dr. Makarian was very persuasive. It did take us about a month, but our company eventually relented and agreed to pre-certify the MRI for coverage, which Shelley subsequently had. While

I suppose we should feel thankful that they changed their minds, the *only* thing they eventually did is what they were ethically obligated to do in the first place. But I suspect most other people in this situation are not so fortunate in coping with such for-profit insurance greed.

A universal, *not*-for-profit healthcare insurance system is not only far more financially efficient than our bloated, costly, for-profit approach, it's successfully used by virtually every other industrialized country in the world. And their populations unmistakably enjoy longer lifespans than those in the U.S.[46] It's the type of coverage already provided for our senior citizens on Medicare. And, nonsensically, government-funded insurance plans are also available for those very politicians who hypocritically vote *against* the public having the same healthcare system they, themselves, use and enjoy. Certainly, even they would agree that no one in this country should ever be faced with having to choose between dying or permanent family financial ruin. I'm *sure* they'd agree. Wouldn't they?

For now, Shelley and I do our best not to focus on the cancer shadow. As we have grown accustomed since diagnosis, we are doing everything we can to take life one day at a time. We'll continue trying not to sweat comparatively small life displeasures while appreciating each day we have, together. Indeed, together is our favorite place to be. Our message to everyone is to consider having a similar outlook and never to take your own good health for granted.

CHAPTER 16

Any Mountain Lion Can Kill You

No amount of guilt can change the past, and no amount of worrying can change the future.

-Umar Ibn Al-Khattaab

I once read a Tumblr.com post by someone calling herself Dread Pirate Khan that made a shrewd analogy comparing her cancer journey to being chased by a mountain lion.[47] The author, who we assume to be female, makes an astute reflection in noting that while she's being stalked by this "godless killing machine," she sees others involved in similar attempted escapes for their own lives. But some of them instead are pursued by smaller mountain lions.

Obviously, this symbolized that their cancers were detected much sooner. Or were less aggressive. Or their disease had responded well to treatment with little in the way of side effects. How unfair it was, she fleetingly thought, that she had a much larger predator hunting her down. Until she noticed yet others being chased by mountain lions far larger and more ferocious than hers, which quickly put her views into a more realistic perspective.

"[Y]ou feel like an asshole for even thinking that," she wrote, "and besides, who in their right mind would want to fight a mountain lion [of any size or shape]?" She quickly understood that while things can *always* be worse, *any* mountain lion can be a killer. Just like cancer.

Cancer fighting is not a competition among those battling the disease. It's anything *but* that. Everyone wants the same outcome in slaying their own mountain lion, regardless of its size. And Shelley recognizes that, as bad as things were, they certainly could have been even worse in comparison to others. Of course, she seldom considers the fact that quite a few things actually *didn't* go her way in treatment, including having to fight her mountain lion in the first place.

As I watch or listen to Shelley interact with other cancer fighters and survivors since her treatment concluded, I can only marvel at the laser-focused connection – the brother- and sisterhood – between and among them. Probably much like war veterans, cancer fighters and survivors share a level of empathy most of us cannot comprehend. Heather M., Heather G., Heather C., Danielle, Kristy, Shea, and others are women in Shelley's circle with past or current experiences in trudging through the long, exhausting gauntlet of various breast cancer treatments. Unlike the rest of us, they can fully grasp the joy of one another's victories and the anguish of their setbacks. And only *they* can truly appreciate and put into perspective their own paths compared with others'. Because of that empathy, the emotional support they feel and can offer one another is immeasurable.

Cancer journeys often vary considerably from one person to the next. The women listed in the previous paragraph shared related diagnoses, but the trails they were forced to forge and subsequently blaze were all different: from different stages and types of their cancer to various treatments to different physical reactions from the same treatments. In addition to offering her endless support and cancer-fighting wisdom, Shelley's emotional responses to her cancer comrades often included an emphasis on how their side effects were sometimes more difficult to manage than hers. Logically, of course, those differences are completely outside of her control and wholly unrelated to her experiences. As I mentioned, cancer fighting is *not* a contest of whoever has it worse somehow wins. While some pathways toward remission are more direct than others, virtually *all* of them are exceedingly difficult, assuming they can be completed in the first place.

Shelley and I were on a walk one afternoon, and I read out loud a text update from Heather G. describing the latest in a series of setbacks stemming from her months-long, ongoing treatment. A relatively young woman in her late 30s, Heather's breast cancer was originally measured at a fairly early stage of 1b. But her cancer type is particularly aggressive. In addition, she suffered from many other serious and ongoing physical maladies prior to her diagnosis ranging from Crohn's Disease to Ehlers-Danlos Syndrome to heart issues, conditions that have been severely tested and exacerbated by her various cancer treatments. Succinctly put, *very* little has gone right for Heather without some sort of major hurdle.

We continued with our walk, and Shelley had a blank expression on her face. About 30 seconds after I finished reading, she softly muttered – perhaps just to herself – "Can't she *ever* catch a break? Why did I get to have it so easy?"

But I heard every word.

While I obviously shared her sentiment about Heather's never-ending bad luck, I was stunned by Shelley's second question. As a front-row spectator to her brutal 14-month series of cancer treatments, I have firsthand observational knowledge that there was *unequivocally nothing* easy about anything she endured in her intense fight. I was so taken aback by what Shelley said that I was momentarily speechless.

Then I finally stopped walking and asked her, "Shelley, do you actually think your cancer fight was *easy*?"

"Well … no, of course not," she quickly backtracked. But, in Shelley's mind, compared to Heather's, it was. "I just sort of feel guilty that she's had a much tougher time of it than I did." And it was that day that I learned about another known side effect of cancer, a psychological one that took place for Shelley after she successfully completed treatment, what many healthcare professionals refer to as a form of *survivor's guilt.*

Survivor's guilt is one of the vast number of complex emotions experienced by cancer fighters and survivors.[48] It is a general mindset that seems to occur to many people surviving some sort of traumatic event – a car crash, a fire, an earthquake, a tornado, or some other natural disaster – that took human life in the process. They may experience guilt in wondering why they were somehow spared when others tragically perished. Apparently it, too, is an extended symptom of PTSD.[49] And it's commonplace among cancer fighters and survivors.

Shelley says she even feels it for cancer fighters she's never met but reads about on social media. Both Shelley and Heather G. have found it to be *very* real in their corresponding cancer worlds.

"I think it's a pretty common reaction," Heather reasoned. "As difficult as my issues have been, I feel the very same way when I meet stage IV cancer patients."

However, she *immediately* reversed course when presented with Shelley's survivor's guilt: "Why would she feel guilty about *me?*" Heather asked. "Her victory is a victory for the whole cancer community, and regardless of my outcome, I *want* Shelley to remain cancer-free and celebrate her victories." For Shelley and Heather, anyway, survivor's guilt seems to be what they feel for cancer fighters who've had things perceptually worse, but apparently they don't want it felt for themselves by others. It's almost as if their empathy sometimes exceeds the reality of their own experiences.

As I further dissect the concept, I suspect that caregivers, too, can feel a strong sense of empathy for one another. Hence, I also have to wonder if there's some sort of secondary or spousal-survivor's guilt. Is it common to feel guilt when my wife somehow survived and others' partners did not? Or is it just me? Why do I feel guilty for their cancer-fighting spouses? Should I not experience it?

Normal or not, I've felt it multiple times not only in my interactions with widowed cancer spouses but with those whose partners are going through rough patches even beyond "normal" cancer horrors. It isn't overwhelming, but it definitely exists for me. As with Shelley's thoughts about Heather, it doesn't seem fair that my wife was finally doing well when others' spouses weren't. But I also know that fairness is but a fantasy and arbitrary portion of one's cancer story. There's really nothing fair about having to fight cancer in the first place. And of course there's also no correlation between Shelley's outcome and others'.

As I look back at my own health issues, I don't recall Shelley telling me she felt any guilt for other cardiac spouses when I survived my lifesaving double-stent procedure to open a couple of blocked arteries several years ago.

I remember talking with others who participated with me in cardiac rehabilitation. They, too, were working their ways back from recent coronary and cardiac issues. I happened to be on a treadmill right next to another individual, a noticeably younger man than I was. Wanting to make conversation to pass the time, I smiled and said, "I know why I'm here. What's *your* story?" He proceeded to tell me that, at the age of 45, he was recovering from his *fourth* heart attack. This one required quadruple-bypass surgery. He said he had a long family history of coronary and cardiac disease. And, my life-threatening blockage notwithstanding, that suddenly put into perspective how relatively easy my stent procedure was compared to his ongoing heart issues.

When I told Shelley about him later that day, her concern seemed exclusively on the fact that my outcome could have been far more serious than it was, and not on my new acquaintance or his wife. As my short-term cardiac caregiver at the time, Shelley certainly didn't indicate that she felt any guilt about my having an easier time than this man or the others in my rehab sessions. She appeared quite happy that everything turned out the way it did in the grand scheme of things, and that I was still with her. No question I feel the same way about Shelley today.

Shelley was near the end of treatment when our good friend Pat passed away after his long battle with cancer. I grieved for him and for his surviving wife, Lucy. It was a cruel fate, one that neither she nor Pat deserved. And I still had my recuperating spouse with me when Lucy no longer did. I confess that I indeed experienced a sense of spousal survivor's guilt. Though I feel it, it still doesn't seem logical. Again, I'm ecstatic to have my healthy wife back, and I wish I could just leave it at that.

Shelley and I both have to remember that one cancer outcome has no random effect on another. If Shelley's health had regressed after Pat's death, it certainly wouldn't have brought him back to Lucy. It would only have meant an increase in overall suffering. And even more so, Pat and Lucy wanted Shelley to beat her cancer regardless of how his battle turned out, just as we wanted Pat to beat his, irrespective of Shelley's overall treatment result.

Therefore, I'm not sure of the usefulness of these guilty feelings. And I don't experience them in other situations. For example, though I feel terrible for those with marital problems, I certainly don't undergo any type of guilt from having a happy marriage. My marriage has nothing to do with theirs. So how does my feeling guilty about Lucy's tragic loss change anything? The answer, of course, is that it doesn't.

As Shelley's post-cancer-treatment successes continue, I feel grateful. I feel blessed. I feel incredibly fortunate. I am overwhelmed with gratitude to those in our cancer clinic. And to our friends who provided help and much needed support in those difficult times. Back in December 2017, I wondered if Shelley would still even be with me in a year. And then to learn, a very long 18 months later with her first post-treatment MRI scan, that her protracted, grueling fight was successful – at least temporarily – was the greatest gift I could ever have received.

I wish for every afflicted cancer fighter and caregiver to experience that sense of cautious triumph. Sadly, it doesn't always happen. Each time we learn of someone's new diagnosis, we feel pain and empathy for them. As others did for Shelley and me, we reach out and try to support them in any conceivable way that we can. And when we hear of someone's heartbreaking death due to cancer, we're devastated for them and their family. I know I'm lucky to still have my wife with me; that she survived to this point the horrors of chemo, surgery, and radiation, and that her oncology team managed to find a way – after hitting more than a couple of brick walls – to get her through everything. And, again, any existence of guilt Shelley or I may feel changes nothing for others.

I also think it's possible Shelley may recently have begun to rethink the "easy" label she put on her treatment in comparison with others. It may be that the passage of time suppresses the memory of cancer-treatment difficulties. After reading the first few chapters in this book about her diagnosis and the specifics of her early and grueling chemotherapy experiences, she said, "I'd forgotten many of the details, and I now realize I probably repressed a lot of those terrible memories."

As a caregiver, I won't venture a guess as to why implicit comparisons to others' more difficult cancer journeys take place and generate these feelings of survivor's guilt. Nonetheless they're real, and, whether or not I fully understand them, downplaying them to anyone would be nothing but unproductive. Logically, I can only hope Shelley and I won't get too emotionally bogged down in contrasting her cancer outcomes with those of others who aren't as fortunate. We do have to accept our feelings as valid, and to perhaps be motivated by them to do something constructive and beneficial as a means of coping with said guilt. But in the end, beating the mountain lion, regardless of size, is every cancer patient's goal. And reaching said goal is nothing to feel guilty about, in spite of differing paths and outcomes others may have.

CHAPTER 17

When Words of Thanks Seem Never to Be Enough

Sometimes you can't pay it back, so you just have to pay it forward.

-Randy Pausch

What do you say to the people who saved your life? Or the life of your spouse? How do you thank them? What words could possibly describe your depth of gratitude? How can you ever pay them back?

Every member of our oncology team at Missouri Cancer Associates played a vital role in our cancer outcome. And when primary treatment was finished, it seemed a little strange, admittedly, not to be maintaining those close relationships we'd developed over the course of more than a year. While they were professional relationships, Shelley and I couldn't help but almost see them as family members.

As I previously wrote, they knew all about us. Obviously about Shelley's cancer fight. About my recent trip to the emergency room for stress-related AFib. Our deep-rooted fears about cancer. Our daughter's wedding. Our son's college graduation. Our professional lives. And we knew of their personal lives as well. We knew who lost her mother to cancer. Who was excited about her new boyfriend. Who was having shoulder surgery. Who liked the same craft breweries, wineries, and coffee houses as did Shelley and I. We laughed together. For goodness sake, we *cried* together. And, perhaps unexpectedly, they also seemed very much to enjoy their interactions with us as well. This, to us, was the very essence of close, personal, if not familial, relationships.

When it came to cancer treatment, these were clearly professional relationships in which the giving and receiving aspects were exclusively – *and by necessity* – one-sided. When friendships seem to materialize between healthcare professionals and patients, the status differential is an obligatory part of the bond, as we were completely dependent on them. Of course, there's a marked difference between those who do their jobs and those who do their jobs well. Treating cancer patients is their *job* – their chosen profession. And our oncology team members seemed quite good at it. While such a profession might be emotionally taxing, they made it clear that they outwardly enjoyed the work they performed. Some of them are even paid handsomely for it. But that doesn't seem to matter if it's you or your spouse whose life has been saved. They are worth every penny and far beyond.

As a college professor, I have the opportunity to establish similarly close, professional relationships with many of my students for one- to four-year periods before they move on. Upon their graduations I'm both happy and sorry to see them go. While I want them to go out and make a difference in the world, of course I will miss them as people when they leave. Some have very graciously told me (whether or not it's actually true) that I was one of their favorite professors because they felt I went the extra mile in helping them throughout their collegiate careers. Others took things a step further by subsequently giving me credit for their successes later in life. And, of course, their words always provide an incredible, touching, feel-good boost to my ego whenever that happens. Rest assured, I am utterly humbled by those wonderful, unsolicited comments.

But all I did was my job – a job I happen to love. It is my profession, and I do it each day to the very best of my ability, regardless of accolades that may or may not follow. Any gratitude students show to their professors during the school year, at commencement, or post-graduation is thick, gooey, sweet icing on top of the cake. For their own sake (and that of their parents and of my institution) *those students have to move on*. All parties win when they graduate and become gainfully employed and independent members of adult society. And then they're replaced by new freshmen and transfers. But, in me, the incoming students get a more seasoned and experienced teacher. And, I would argue, a *better* teacher because of those experiences with the students of the past. So without their even trying, that is a significant way graduates of my institution have paid me back.

When Shelley got better, it was time for us to move on too. We had to leave our superb oncology staff so they could provide their lifesaving skills and services to others just beginning their own fights against cancer. But the skills and services they'll offer actually won't be the same. They'll be even better because of the added experiences they had with Shelley and those who were simultaneously treated along with her.

But not everyone gets a happy ending to their cancer story. People like my father may die from their cancer. Dad fought through so many horrors in his years of treatment, which, ultimately, did not save his life. A few days before he passed, I thanked him not only for being the greatest father and role model I could possibly have had, but also for continuing to fight what was inevitably an unwinnable war for as long and hard as he did. I asked him if he felt a trade-off of his terrible side effects was worth the possibility of just a little more time. His answer was a profound surprise to me: "No," he said, "but I'm not doing this for myself. I only survived cancer as long as I have because others before me took their chances with new treatments. Even if I don't make it, my doctors can still learn from my illness."

Aside from being a brilliant academic scholar and teacher, Dad was the most noble and selfless individual I've ever known. And he knew that acquiring the knowledge of what didn't work to treat his cancer was every bit as critical to medical science as learning what did. He was right of course. In the spirit of Thomas Edison, who was purported to have said, "I have not failed. I have just found 10,000 ways that won't work,"[50] my father trudged forward. He kept going, even when hope was all but lost, and *that's how he gave back*. Oncologists treat us and often save us. But either way they learn from us. And by virtue of our very participation in the cancer treatment process, we *do* teach them in return. And they become better for it.

As Shelley's adjuvant treatment continues, we'll still see the MCA crowd, but only once every few months at most, which is quite unlike the weekly and even daily contact during much of her chemo and radiation. We have certainly missed them as people, but not as professionals. Unless, God forbid, we need them again in the future because of a recurrence.

But I guess it does bring us back to the original question: When cancer treatment has been successfully completed, how do you appropriately thank your oncology team? I. Don't. Know. Perhaps with a floral arrangement, a gift certificate, a coffee club membership, a plate of brownies, a bottle of fine whiskey, or a greeting card. Or … maybe just tell them in person or write an individual letter to each member of your staff to simply say *thank you*: Thank you for saving me. For saving my partner. For helping to make the worst of human situations tolerable, livable, and, eventually, much better. Thank you for listening. Thank you for caring far beyond what your professional obligations could ever require. And, most of all, *thank you for being so damn good at your job*.

Though thankful words will *never* seem to be enough, my experience, when I'm the one on the receiving end, is that they're probably *far* more powerful than you could ever imagine.

Shelley and I would love to find a more tangible way give back what we received, but it may not be possible in the oncology world. Of course we have made, and will continue to make, repeated donations to a variety of reputable cancer research organizations. And though that's important, it doesn't seem quite as personal. So in terms of "giving" or "paying back," I wonder if it might be more appropriate and realistic to simply replace the word "back" with "forward."

Just as our cancer-surviving/fighting friends did for Shelley and me at the outset of our battle by showing indispensable empathy and compassion and holding us up with their support, Shelley and I can do the same for others. Those who are about to begin their personal horror stories are entering the dark and treacherous cave of cancer and its treatment. Perhaps we can at least give them a metaphorical flashlight to partially illuminate their new, frightening surroundings by sharing our experiences with them. By imparting our stories, we can give them a little bit of hope and predictability, which is what we found to be so useful.

And when they finish their arduous journeys, they can do the same for the next unlucky cancer families. Because until we have at our disposal more than 100 different cures, those families will keep coming, replacing both the survivors and the fallen. We may never be able to pay it *back*, but we can certainly pay it *forward*. We'll continue to do that for the rest of our lives. And that's the way it should be.

And finally, as I conclude this personal cancer caregiving book with a lesson on thank-yous, I need to communicate a special, public thanks to my beautiful wife:

> Shelley, thank you for your everlasting love, and for your grit and determination throughout this ordeal. You were the one constant. The oncology team was paramount; our friends, neighbors, and co-workers were vital. In their supportive social media posts, many readers attributed credit for your recovery to a multitude of scientific and spiritual directions.

But the reality is that you are entitled to *all* of the credit. You were the one who had to tolerate *everything*. The most difficult thing I've ever had to do was watch you suffer as you have. You never deserved any of this crap. But you not only did it without complaining, you kept up a perpetually positive image. I suspect many who were watching you often thought you never missed a beat in the rhythm of life (although we both know *far* better than that). And though I'm sorry you had to show me in this manner, you are indeed the strongest and most beautiful individual I've ever known. When you lost your hair, when you were frail and your face turned ashen, you *still* were able to smile at me. Even under those horrific circumstances, I never saw anything more stunning than your irrepressible spirit shoving aside the physical infirmities to brightly shine through. I'm in absolute awe of you. You are my hero and the love of my life. The greatest decision I ever made was when I asked you to be my life partner. And the greatest thing that ever happened to me was when you said "Yes." In you, I truly won the marriage lottery. Darling, I love you infinitely. I've absolutely cherished our first 30+ years together. And I hope we have 30 more.

Invictus, Baby!

Endnotes

1   Monarth, H. The irresistible power of storytelling as a strategic business tool. *Harvard Business Review*. 3/11/14. https://hbr.org/2014/03/the-irresistible-power-of-storytelling-as-a-strategic-business-tool

2   American Cancer Society. Cancer Facts & Figures 2020. https://www.cancer.org/research/cancer-facts-statistics/all-cancer-facts-figures/cancer-facts-figures-2020.html

3   '1 in 2 people will develop cancer in their lifetime'. *Medical News Today*. https://www.medicalnewstoday.com/articles/288916

4   Mandell, A. Julia Louis-Dreyfus: 'One in eight women get breast cancer; today, I'm the one'. *USA Today*, 9/28/17. https://www.usatoday.com/story/life/people/2017/09/28/julia-louis-dreyfus-reveals-breast-cancer-diagnosis-pushes-universal-healthcare/713156001/

5   Aitkenhead, A. Siddhartha Mukherjee: 'A positive attitude does not cure cancer, any more than a negative one causes it.' The Guardian. 12/2011https://www.theguardian.com/books/2011/dec/04/siddhartha-mukherjee-talk-about-cancer

6   National Cancer Institute. What is cancer? https://www.cancer.gov/about-cancer/understanding/what-is-cancer#types

7   American Cancer Society. What is cancer? https://www.cancer.org/cancer/cancer-basics/what-is-cancer.html

8   Peters, C.C. A thing about cancer, *Boulevard*. https://boulevardmagazine.org/clinton-crockett-peters

9   Shariff-Marco, S., Klassen, A. C., and Bowie, J.V. Racial/Ethnic differences in self-reported racism and its association with cancer-related health behaviors. *American Journal of Public Health*. 2/2010. https://ajph.aphapublications.org/doi/full/10.2105/AJPH.2009.163899

10   'Jeopardy!' host Alex Trebek opens up about cancer battle | GMA. YouTube. 5/1/19. https://www.youtube.com/watch?v=_ILNc6Qpjwc&feature=youtu.be

11   DeVito, J.A. *The interpersonal communication book*. 14th ed. Pearson, 2016. p. 264.

12   Center for Disease Control Prevention, mortality in the United States, 2017. *National Center for Health Statistics, Data Brief No. 328, November 2018.* https://www.cdc.gov/nchs/products/databriefs/db328.htm

13   Rousy, K. Cancer lingo: How one person's thoughtful metaphor can be another's cliché. *CBC News.* 8/13/17. https://www.cbc.ca/news/health/cancer-methaphors-cliches-mccain-language-sunnybrook-mountsinai-1.4241058

14   Glorioso, A. I'm coping with cancer by reporting on it. *Politico.* 8/19/18. https://www.politico.com/magazine/story/2018/08/19/im-coping-with-cancer-by-reporting-on-it-219372

15   National Breast Cancer Foundation. Breast Cancer Stages. 2019. https://www.nationalbreastcancer.org/about-breast-cancer/breast-cancer-staging

16   Cancer.net. What to expect when having chemotherapy. 6/2019. https://www.cancer.net/navigating-cancer-care/how-cancer-treated/chemotherapy/what-expect-when-having-chemotherapy

17   Reviewed by Waks, A.G. AC: Adriamycin and Cyclophosphamide. *Living Beyond Breast Cancer.* https://www.lbbc.org/learn/treatments-and-research/chemotherapy/common-chemotherapy-regimens/ac-adriamycin-and

18   Caldwell, E. A satisfying romantic relationship may improve breast cancer survivors' health. *Science Magazine.* 6/2/20. https://scienmag.com/a-satisfying-romantic-relationship-may-improve-breast-cancer-survivors-health/

19   https://www.treasurequotes.com/quotes/shared-joy-is-a-double-joy-shared-sorrow-is-h

20   Parisella, J. Civility is not a sign of weakness. *Americas Quarterly.* 8/18/12. https://www.americasquarterly.org/civility-is-not-a-sign-of-weakness

21   American Cancer Society. Getting help for chemo brain. 6/2017. https://www.cancer.org/content/dam/cancer-org/cancer-control/en/booklets-flyers/getting-help-for-chemo-brain-english.pdf

22   https://www.goodreads.com/quotes/447645-an-apology-is-the-superglue-of-life-it-can-repair

23   Hardeman, K.T. When your partner has breast cancer: some (not so) obvious caregiving tips from a husband's perspective. *Coping with Cancer.* September/October 2019. https://www.copingmag.com/coping-with-cancer/when-your-partner-has-breast-cancer

24   From the Michael Franks album *Time Together*

25   Breastcancer.org. Post-Traumatic Stress Disorder (PTSD). https://www.breastcancer.org/treatment/side_effects/stress_disorder

26   Cancer.net editorial board. Post-traumatic stress disorder and cancer. 3/2019. https://www.cancer.net/survivorship/life-after-cancer/post-traumatic-stress-disorder-and-cancer

27   https://doncharisma.org/2020/04/13/worrying-doesnt-stop-the-bad-stuff-from-happening-it-just-stops-you-from-enjoying-the-good-stuff-karen-salmansohn/

28   https://www.imdb.com/title/tt0088247/characters/nm0000299

29   Gehlert, H. Navigating relationships amid a cancer diagnosis. CaringBridge. 7/28/2020 https://www.caringbridge.org/visit/heathergehlert

30   The Esteé Lauder companies' new book encourages women to reflect on life beyond breast cancer. *Marie Claire*. 10/21/15. https://www.marieclaire.co.uk/news/beauty-news/estee-lauder-campaign-breast-cancer-quotes-37968

31   Finn, N. The truth about Michael J. Fox and Tracy Pollan's inspiring 30-year love story. *E! News*. 7/16/19. https://www.eonline.com/news/951505/the-truth-about-michael-j-fox-and-tracy-pollan-s-inspiring-30-year-love-story

32   American Cancer Society. How common Is breast cancer? 9/18/19. https://www.cancer.org/cancer/breast-cancer/about/how-common-is-breast-cancer.html

33   Brody J.E. The shock of lung cancer, when it strikes nonsmokers. *The New York Times*. 3/21/06. https://www.nytimes.com/2006/03/21/health/21brody.html

34   Whittington, E. Medical miracle or spontaneous remission?: What are the odds that some cancers spontaneously go into remission? https://www.curetoday.com/publications/cure/2007/spring2007/Medical-Miracle-or-Spontaneous-Remission

35   Aitkenhead, A. Siddhartha Mukherjee: 'A positive attitude does not cure cancer, any more than a negative one causes it.' The Guardian. 12/2011. https://www.theguardian.com/books/2011/dec/04/siddhartha-mukherjee-talk-about-cancer

36   Aitkenhead, A. Siddhartha Mukherjee: 'A positive attitude does not cure cancer, any more than a negative one causes it.' The Guardian. 12/2011. https://www.theguardian.com/books/2011/dec/04/siddhartha-mukherjee-talk-about-cancer

37   Aitkenhead, A. Siddhartha Mukherjee: 'A positive attitude does not cure cancer, any more than a negative one causes it.' *The Guardian*. 12/2011. https://www.theguardian.com/books/2011/dec/04/siddhartha-mukherjee-talk-about-cancer

38   Mayo Clinic. Radiation therapy for breast cancer. https://www.mayoclinic.org/tests-procedures/radiation-therapy-for-breast-cancer/about/pac-20384940

39   Breastcancer.org. The radiation planning session (simulation). 5/30/13. https://www.breastcancer.org/treatment/radiation/types/ext/expect/simulation

40 Breastcancer.org. Myths about radiation therapy. 6/20/16. https://www.breastcancer.org/treatment/radiation/myths

41 Mayo Clinic. Capecitabine (Oral Route). 5/1/2020. https://www.mayoclinic.org/drugs-supplements/capecitabine-oral-route/side-effects/drg-20062501?p=1

42 Mitchell, J. I'm done with cancer treatment. Why am I so upset all the time? *Coping with Cancer*. September/October 2018. https://www.copingmag.com/coping-with-cancer/i-m-done-with-cancer-treatment-why-am-i-so-upset-all-the-time

43 Smith, S. Surviving cancer puts you at risk for PTSD. *Coping with Cancer*. November/December 2019. https://www.copingmag.com/coping-with-cancer/surviving-cancer-puts-you-at-risk-for-ptsd

44 Fitzpatrick, T. The financial impact of a cancer diagnosis. *Cancer Support Community*. 2/7/18. https://www.cancersupportcommunity.org/blog/2018/02/financial-impact-cancer-diagnosis

45 https://www.quotes.net/quote/3138

46 Saleh, N. Why the US has lower life expectancy than other countries *MDLinx*. 2/15/2020. https://www.mdlinx.com/article/why-the-us-has-lower-life-expectancy-than-other-countries/70SKTKpuQRVJJ0rmIckYrH

47 Dread Pirate Khan. *tumblr*. 4/30/15. https://dreadpiratekhan.tumblr.com/post/117758401541/whats-it-like-to-go-through-cancer-treatment

48 Willingsham, S. The secret side effect of survivorship: survivor's guilt. *Cure*. 11/11/19. https://www.curetoday.com/publications/heal/2019/fall-2019/the-secret-side-effect-of-survivorship-survivors-guilt

49 Cherry, K. Understanding survivor's guilt. *Verywell Mind*. 2/26/20. https://www.verywellmind.com/survivors-guilt-4688743

50 Quote Investigator. https://quoteinvestigator.com/2012/07/31/edison-lot-results/

CPSIA information can be obtained
at www.ICGtesting.com
Printed in the USA
LVHW012056220921
698519LV00004B/55